An Atlas of
CONTRACEPTION

THE ENCYCLOPEDIA OF VISUAL MEDICINE SERIES

An Atlas of CONTRACEPTION

Pramilla Senanayake
IPPF, Regent's College, London, UK

and

Malcolm Potts
University of California,
Berkeley, USA

The Parthenon Publishing Group
International Publishers in Medicine, Science & Technology

NEW YORK LONDON

British Library Cataloguing in Publication Data
Senanayake, Pramilla
Atlas of Contraception. – (Encyclopedia of Visual Medicine Series)
I. Title II. Potts, D. M. III. Series
613.94
ISBN 1-85070-387-6

Library of Congress Cataloging-in-Publication Data
Senanayake, Pramilla.
An atlas of contraception/ P. Senanayake and D. M. Potts.
p. cm. – (The Encyclopedia of visual medicine series)
Includes bibliographical references and index.
ISBN 1-85070-387-6
I. Contraception. 2. Contraceptives. 3. Contraception–Atlases. 4. Contraceptives–Atlases.
I. Potts, Malcolm. II. Title. III. Series.
[DNLM: I. Contraception–atlases. 2. Contraception Agents–atlases. 3. Contraception Devices–atlases. WP 17 S474a 1994]

RG 136.S46 1994
613.9'4–dc20
DNLM/DLC
for Library of Congress 94-12891
CIP

Published in the UK and Europe by
The Parthenon Publishing Group Limited
Casterton Hall, Carnforth
Lancs. LA6 2LA

Published in North America by
The Parthenon Publishing Group Inc.
One Blue Hill Plaza
PO Box 1564, Pearl River
New York 10965, USA

First published 1995

Typeset by AMA Graphics Limited, Preston
Printed and bound by TG Hostench S.A., Spain

Contents

The Encyclopedia of Visual Medicine Series

Titles currently planned in this series include:

An Atlas of Oncology
An Atlas of Hypertension
An Atlas of Common Diseases
An Atlas of Osteoporosis
An Atlas of the Menopause
An Atlas of Contraception
An Atlas of Endometriosis
An Atlas of Ultrasonography in Obstetrics and Gynecology
An Atlas of Practical Radiology
An Atlas of Psoriasis
An Atlas of Trauma Management
An Atlas of Lung Infections
An Atlas of Transvaginal Color Doppler
An Atlas of Infective Endocarditis
An Atlas of Rheumatology
An Atlas of Epilepsy
An Atlas of Differential Diagnosis in HIV Disease
An Atlas of Practical Dermatology
An Atlas of Laser Operative Laparoscopy and Hysteroscopy
An Atlas of Atherosclerosis
An Atlas of Eye Diseases
An Atlas of Cutaneous Growths
An Atlas of Myocardial Infarction
An Atlas of Diabetes Mellitus

Preface

Over the past two decades, family planning has become recognized as a medical specialty with professional organizations, peer-reviewed journals and national and international meetings. It was not always so. There could not have been an atlas of this type in 1950, and even in 1980 it might have looked very different.

Family planning is a branch of preventive medicine which can have a profound impact on the health of women and their children. Like many other aspects of medicine, certain contraceptive choices require surgical or clinical skills in order to be used correctly. For some couples with chronic sickness or inheritable diseases, family planning advice is an intrinsic part of comprehensive patient care. Physicians have also taken a leadership role in family planning because they often see the acute suffering that occurs when people are denied family planning choices. At the same time, family planning differs from other branches of medicine in two critical ways: it is only successful when those concerned recognize that family planning involves consumer choices more than physician prescriptions and in most cases it deals with healthy people. It must be recognized that, though some contraceptives have been developed by medical researchers, the actual distribution of these methods i.e. getting the right contraceptive to the right individual at the right place and right cost, involves many groups of service providers, the majority of them being non-clinical. The tension between consumer choices and conventional clinical perspectives is especially strong in the case of abortion. In putting this atlas together we have tried to keep these several perspectives in mind and, in order to better understand today's issues, we have also noted some of the history of family planning.

We are grateful to colleagues who have provided material and to The Parthenon Publishing Group and Gill Hardy, the volume editor, for their patience and attention to detail. But above all we are grateful to the women and men all over the world who it has been our privilege to care for and who, in turn, have taught us the things we now know about this specialty. One thing we are certain about: family planning will continue to evolve and it will continue to remain important to hundreds of millions of people in all nations and of every background.

Pramilla Senanayake
Malcolm Potts

1

Introduction

Reproduction is a lifelong process, not merely the passion of sexual intercourse or the pain of childbirth. It begins when the germ cells (which give rise to ova and sperm) are set aside early in embryonic life, and is still continuing when the grandparents do the baby-sitting. Medical science has been able to interrupt, or to devise potential new methods of contraception, at most steps in the long process from the formation of eggs and sperm to the fertilization of the egg, its attachment to the uterus and the early embryonic development. Figure 1.1 shows the points in the process at which fertility can be controlled through intervention.

Family planning is wanted, simple and inexpensive. It also involves areas of human sexuality which are perceived to be controversial and where public attitudes are conservative. The technologies which exist for the artificial control of human fertility need to be reviewed from two very different perspectives. The first is that of normal, healthy reproductive physiology; the second is that of public policy-making in an area of private concern.

Health professionals have a central role to play in family planning for two differing reasons. First, their work often gives them insight into private and intimate problems that individuals may be reluctant to share with others; and, second, they have technical skills that are essential for the proper use of several – although by no means all – methods of fertility regulation.

It is easy to forget that human beings are the slowest breeding mammals known. Puberty occurs later than in any other species, and pregnancies are naturally spaced by long intervals of infertility associated with lactation. In addition, we are the only species with a clear-cut menopause followed by many years of infertile life in the female. In the few preliterate hunter–gatherer societies that are relatively untouched by the modern world, such as the !Khun from the Kalahari desert or the Gangi from the highlands of New Guinea, puberty does not occur until the late teens or even early twenties. Babies are suckled on demand for 2 or 3 years and breastfeeding leads to the suppression of ovulation for 1–2 years. As a result, in the absence of any knowledge of contraception, pregnancies in preliterate societies are naturally spaced 3 or 4 years apart. Women in such societies commonly have only four to six live-born children in a lifetime; approximately half of these children die from childhood diseases and accidents before they themselves can reproduce. Thus, the population of the Kalahari !Khun doubles approximately every 300 years.

By contrast, in a modern society the age of puberty has fallen (probably as a result of nutritional changes). Patterns of breastfeeding have changed or the practice has been entirely replaced by bottle feeding: the technology of milk formula and prepared infant foods has had a remarkable effect on human fertility. In the absence of breastfeeding, a woman may have eight to ten live-born children in a lifetime. At the same time, a miraculous and welcome decline in infant mortality has occurred. The result: the population in a country such as contemporary Kenya doubles every 18 years. Worldwide, human beings now number 5.6 billion and are increasing by 1 million every 4 days (Figure 1.2).

These changes have not only had a marked impact on potential family size, but they have also had a catastrophically adverse effect on the health of individual women. Frequent childbearing, particularly amongst teenagers and women over the age of 35 years, greatly increases the risk of mortality and ill health among the women concerned. Less visible, but equally important, changes in the age of puberty (Figures 1.3 and 1.4) and in patterns of childbearing have been associated with an increased incidence of a number of diseases, particularly reproductive cancers. It is estimated that cancer of the breast is 120 times more common in Western women than in hunter–gatherer societies.

Early menarche, late menopause and late first full-term pregnancy are three risk factors for breast cancer (Figure 1.5).

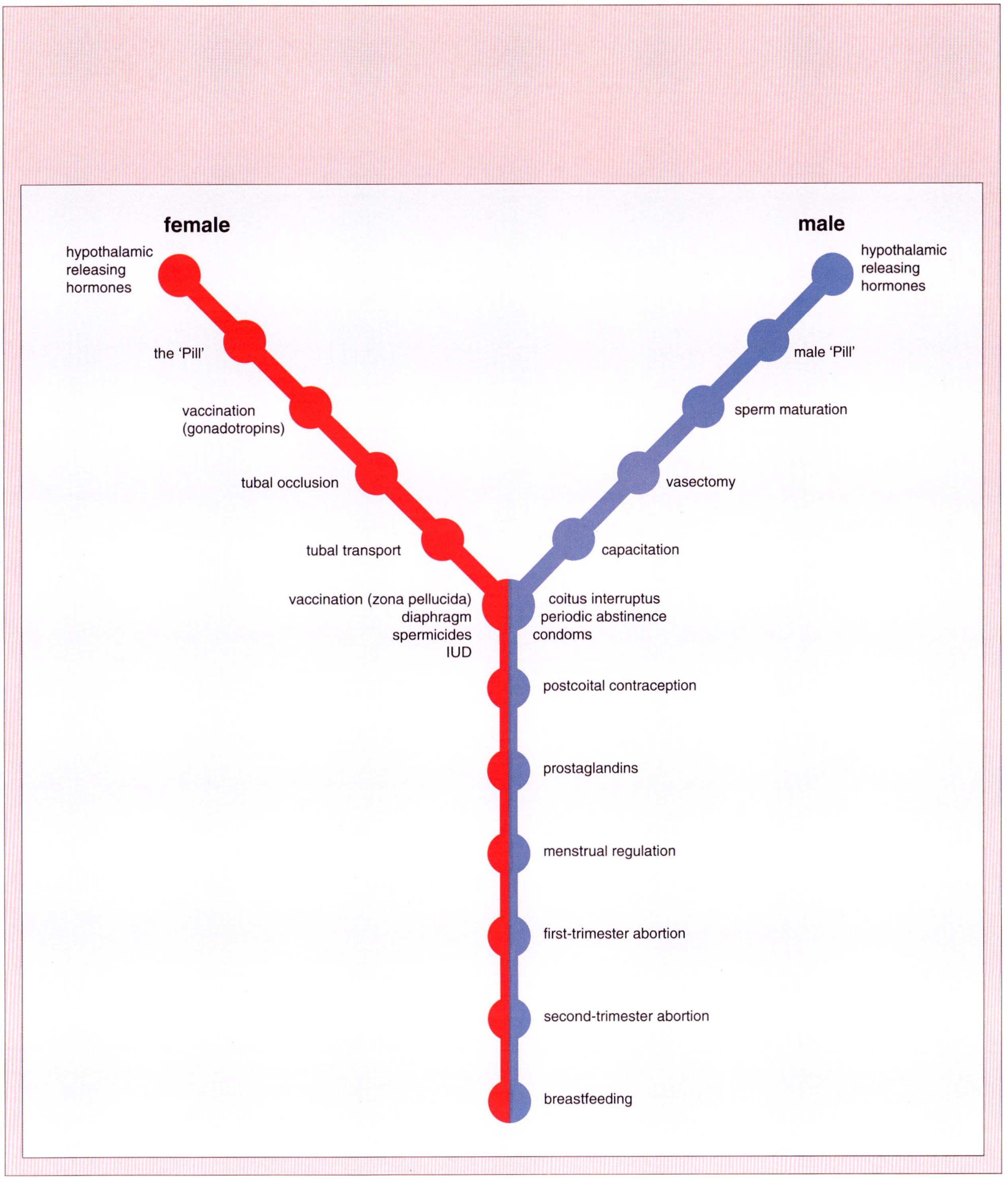

Figure 1.1 The chart shows possible points of intervention to control fertility both up to and after the point of fertilization (not all the possibilities mentioned above are available in practice)

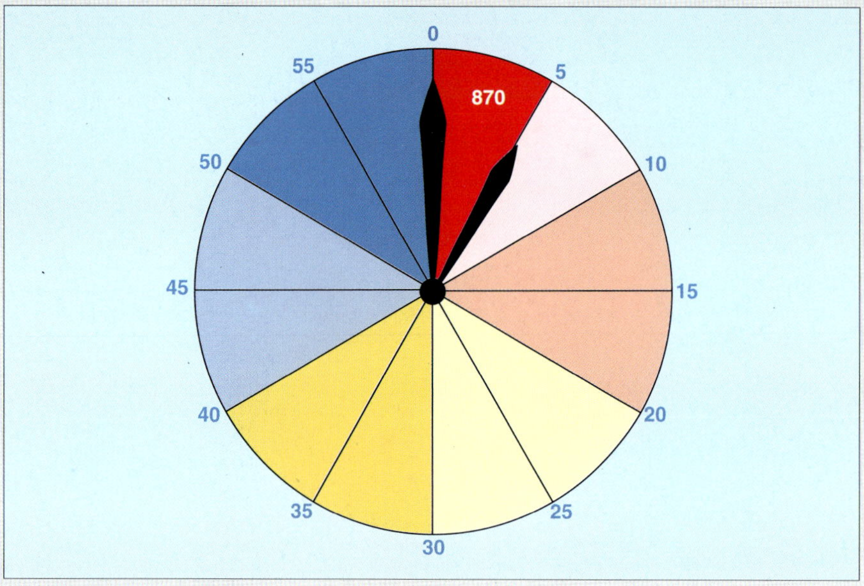

Figure 1.2 Rate of worldwide population increase. Worldwide, the population is increasing by 1 million every 4 days (i.e. by 870 every 5 minutes)

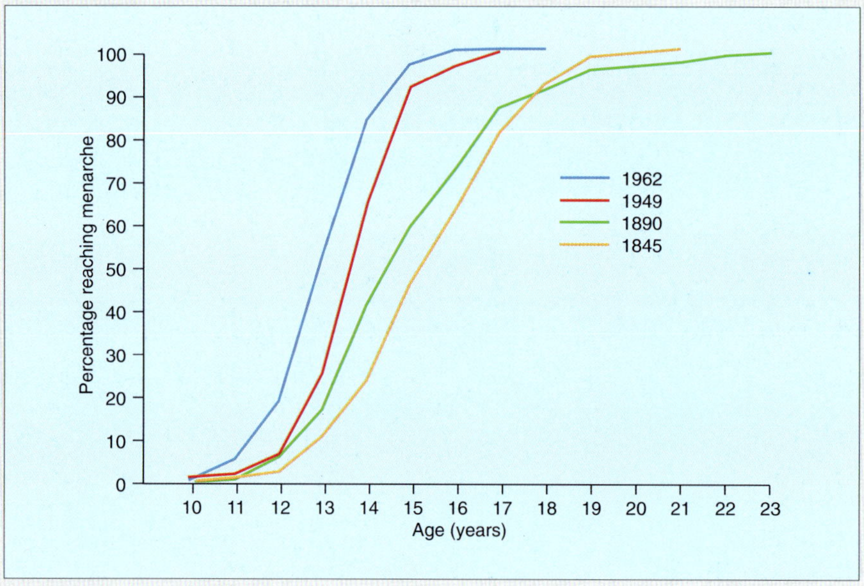

Figure 1.3 Changes in the age of menarche in England. In 1962, 50% of girls had started to menstruate by 13 years of age. A century earlier the corresponding figure was a little over 15 years. Also, as shown by the slope of the curve, the variation was greater in the nineteenth century, from 11 years to 19 years compared with 10–16 years for girls in the 1960s. (Adapted from Parkes, A. S. (1976). *Patterns of Sexuality and Reproduction*, p. 18. (Oxford: Oxford University Press))

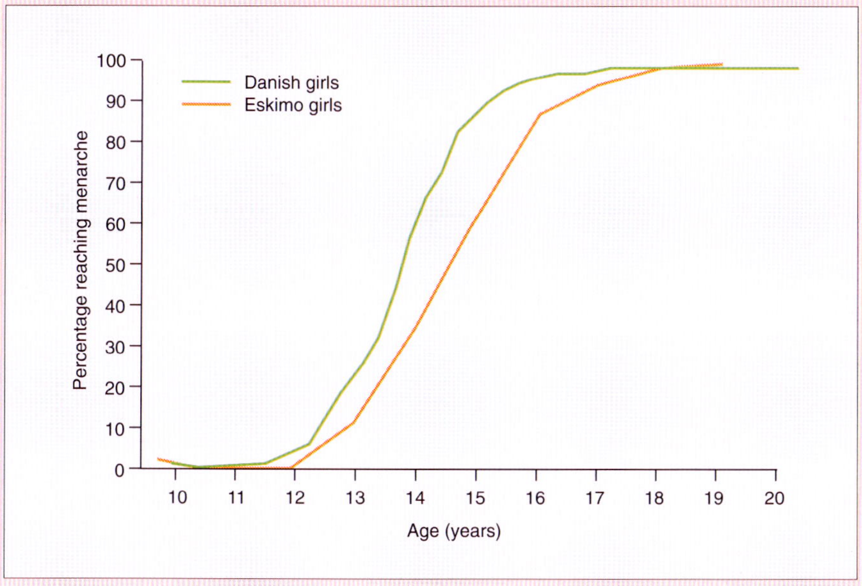

Figure 1.4 Age at menarche among the Eskimos in Southwest Greenland compared with that of Danish girls in Copenhagen. Eskimo girls are about 2 years older than Danish ones at the stage when 50% are menstruating. (Adapted from Parkes, A. S. (1970). *Patterns of Sexuality and Reproduction*, p. 19. (Oxford: Oxford University Press))

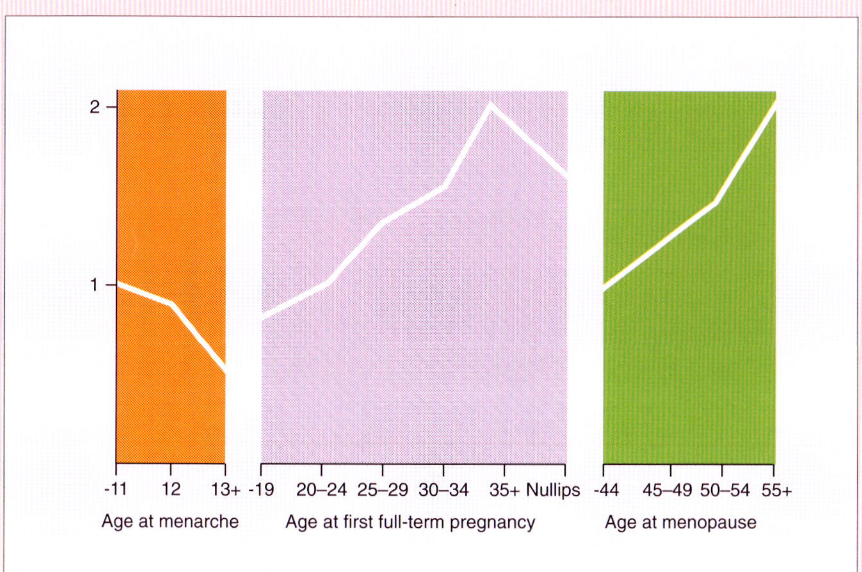

Figure 1.5 Relative risks for breast cancer

2

Rationale for family planning

Reproduction in animals is characterized by a vast overproduction of sperm and eggs and a high degree of wastage of early pregnancy. A single human ejaculate represents more potential human beings than are found in the whole of the southern USA and central America (Figure 2.1). A healthy man in his lifetime produces enough sperm to replace the whole human race. It is estimated that 114 million acts of sexual intercourse take place each day resulting in 910 000 conceptions and 356 000 sexually transmitted bacterial and viral infections.

Early in embryonic life a woman has 6 million eggs, each genetically unique, in her ovaries. Most of these are lost before puberty; only a few hundred will be ovulated in her lifetime (Figure 2.2) and usually well under twenty will be fertilized (Figure 2.3). Many eggs and sperm have obvious microscopic defects and special studies show that chromosomal and other less visible abnormalities are even more common (Figure 2.4). Approximately half the eggs fertilized are naturally wasted even before a woman is aware that a pregnancy has taken place. Once a woman's period is late and pregnancy is recognized, up to 30% of embryos will still go on to abort spontaneously. The overwhelming majority of these early losses are of defective embryos that would not have survived to delivery, or if they did, would have produced grossly abnormal babies. Figure 2.5 illustrates the rate of spontaneous abortions by duration of pregnancy.

In addition to this natural wastage, maternal and social factors contribute to the risk involved in any pregnancy. Family planning has a significant role to play in minimizing this risk for the individuals. The more people are helped to implement their personal choices about family size, the slower will be the growth in world population.

HEALTH RATIONALE

High-risk pregnancies

Birth planning can prevent high-risk pregnancies. The risk of maternal or infant morbidity and mortality is the highest in four specific types of pregnancies. In situations where maternal nutrition is not a problem and where good and regular antenatal, delivery and postnatal care are available, these risks may be somewhat reduced. The four high-risk groups are:

(1) Too young – maternal age less than 18 years;

(2) Too old – after age 35 years;

(3) Too many – after four births; and

(4) Too close – less than 2 years apart.

Figure 2.6 shows how these factors interact.

Mothers too early

Globally, the percentage of women marrying under

20 years of age varies (Figure 2.7) and 10–15% of live births are to teenagers (Figures 2.8 and 2.9). This has both social (educational, emotional and financial) and biological (prematurity, low birth weight, malnutrition and infection) consequences. Adolescent mothers are at greater risk of toxemia, anemia, miscarriage and obstetric complications. Their offspring are at increased risk of prematurity, infant mortality and congenital abnormalities (Figure 2.10).

The child of multiple risks faces even greater problems. For example, a child born to a teenage mother less than 2 years after an earlier child faces an additional 116% risk of death before the age of 1 year if the previous child survived; if the previous child died, that additional risk rises to 320%.

Mothers too late

Late pregnancy also involves additional risk to mother and child. Figure 2.11 shows the percentage of all children born to women over 35 years of age in a number of countries.

Too many children

In terms of risks and complications, the optimal number of children for a woman to bear is two or three. Pregnancies occurring after four births are associated with increased risks to both the mother and child (Figures 2.12 and 2.13). Serious complications of pregnancy and delivery including hemorrhage, infection and toxemia are more likely, as is anemia. The child faces the possibility of malnutrition due to increased family size , and is more likely to suffer from infectious illnesses, to have reduced physical growth and development, and less than optimal school performance.

Too close together

Pregnancies less than 2 years apart also pose increased risks to both mother and child. Frequent pregnancies cause a drain on the mother's nutritional status, and she may develop a maternal depletion syndrome. The child may have low birth weight and may suffer from malnutrition and poor health, as well as reduced physical growth and development, and decreased academic achievement. Figure 2.14 shows the infant and child mortality rates according to spacing of pregnancies. Figure 2.15 shows measures of intelligence and growth with respect to birth interval among children in Singapore.

As well as the increased likelihood of physical and intellectual problems, frequent births result in the mother devoting less time to each young child (Figure 2.16).

Maternal mortality/morbidity

Figure 2.17 shows the estimated annual number of maternal deaths in various parts of the world. Maternal mortality rates vary from five to 30/100 000 live births in developed countries to 50–800/100 000 in developing countries. In the USA, less than one out of 100 deaths are of women in their child-bearing years. This rises to one out of four deaths in developing countries. Figure 2.18 correlates female life expectancy and total fertility rates in various countries. The causes of maternal mortality include obstetric factors, health service factors, low rates of contraceptive use and low socioeconomic status. Obstetric factors include hemorrhage, infection, toxemia, obstructed labor and unsafe induced abortion. Health service factors which contribute to maternal mortality are lack of availability of treatment for complications, shortage of staff and supplies, and improper treatment.

Low rates of contraceptive use result in uncontrolled child-bearing, which in turn exposes high-risk women to the dangers of pregnancy. A woman's lifetime chance of maternal death accumulates, so that each pregnancy further increases the risk. Unwanted pregnancies prompt 'back street' abortions, which result in injury and maternal deaths.

Low socioeconomic status often entails a lack of access to health care. In addition, malnutrition and a low social status of women contribute to maternal mortality.

A number of measures can be taken to reduce maternal mortality. Provision of family planning services, provision of obstetric first aid at health centers and rural maternity centers, upgrading of rural hospitals, expansion of the role of midwives, nurses and medical assistants, establishment of maternity waiting homes, and community education all are of benefit in improving maternal health and reducing mortality. For example, Sri Lanka and Pakistan have the same gross national product, but the maternal mortality rate in Sri Lanka is one-fifth that of Pakistan; almost all births in Sri Lanka are attended by trained health personnel, and there are good family planning services and high female literacy.

Infant and child mortality/morbidity

In developing countries today, about 5.6 million infant deaths and 200 000 maternal deaths could be avoided if family planning choices and obstetric care were improved.

Child health problems related to high-risk pregnancy include low birth weight, poor childhood nutrition, more frequent episodes of infectious diseases, slower physical growth and development, a higher risk of congenital abnormalities, and reduced intellectual performance. Anything which reduces a child's potential in life is an obscene thing – and lack of family planning is all too often just such a barrier to child development.

HUMAN RIGHTS/REPRODUCTIVE RIGHTS RATIONALE

Over the last quarter of a century, the ability of individuals to choose the number and spacing of their children has been recognized as a basic human right. According to the World Population Plan of Action, 'All individuals and couples have the right to decide freely and responsibly the number and spacing of their children and to have the information, education and the means to do so; the responsibility of couples and individuals in the exercise of this right takes into account the needs of their living and future children and their responsibilities towards the community' (Mexico City, 1984).

Individual world leaders and international meetings in Tehran (1968) and Mexico City (1984), as well as a number of declarations on human rights by the United Nations, all place an obligation on governments to offer their citizens family planning choices. Unfortunately, a gap remains between political rhetoric and practical choices. Many individuals in the Third World simply do not have access to family planning information and services. Often particular methods of family planning are not permitted or there are arbitrary limitations on access to voluntary surgical contraception and abortion.

The eroding status of low-income women in developing countries is a base-line indicator of human progress. Ignoring this issue is not only untenable, it is in the long run self-defeating. The health risks of poverty are far greater for females than for males. Policy measures for sustainable development must be accompanied by concrete actions towards the improvement of health, nutrition, sanitation and access to safe water. In addition, effective family planning programs must be in place. If a woman is unable to control her fertility, it is unlikely that she will have control over the other aspects of her life.

DEVELOPMENT RATIONALE

For a thousand centuries following the evolution of our species, parents, on average, could expect to see two children survive and reproduce in the next generation, even though they might have delivered four to six babies. If this was not true, the 'population explosion' would have happened a long time ago. Then for about 100 years in the West and 50 years in the developing world, a rapid fall in infant mortality and changes in breastfeeding patterns that increased fertility, suddenly meant that four to six children were surviving until the next generation. As a result, the global population has doubled at shorter and shorter intervals.

According to the US National Academy of Sciences 1986 Report, the world as a whole is in transition. Fertility has fallen to 48% of the birth rates found after the Second World War to family sizes which would be compatible with a stable global population. In some developing countries where good family planning services have been made available, the birth rate has fallen two to four times as rapidly as it did in the West at a similar stage of the demographic transition (Figure 2.19).

The declining fertility in Western Europe and North America in the nineteenth and twentieth centuries was almost certainly seriously retarded by lack of access to contraceptive choices. Hospital records for women admitted for complications of illegal abortion in the first half of the twentieth century are a testimony to the innumerable desperate attempts made by women to restrict family size.

There is a consistent relationship between the birth rate and the use of contraceptives. For every 15% rise in contraceptive prevalence, the average number of children in a family falls by one. Wherever contraceptives have been readily available, and particularly where safe abortion services have been accessible, fertility has fallen rapidly. There was a time when demographers argued that there were intrinsic differences in desired family size between various social, economic and religious groups. In practice, wherever the barriers to fertility regulation have been removed, differences in various groups have disappeared. This is well illustrated by the history of Protestant and Catholic groups in the United States since 1950: for a while, Catholic fertility was consistently higher than Protestant, but once contraceptives became acceptable and widely available and abortion was legalized, the differences disappeared. Interestingly, there is little or no difference in the percentage of women of different religious groups who resort to abortion (Figure 2.20).

THE POPULATION EXPLOSION

How long will it take for the second half of the global demographic transition to be completed? Until approximately 10 000 years ago, the world population was no more than 5 million. The transition from hunting–gathering to settled agriculture meant that many more people could be supported by the same area of land. The result was a gradual increase in the population which reached about 200 million by the time of Christ. By 1987, the world population had exceeded 5 billion. This landmark shows the unprecedented rate of growth of the human population. The first billion was not reached until 1830. It then took 100 years to reach the second billion, but only 45 years to double again to 4 billion in 1975. It is estimated that the 6 billion mark will be reached by 1998 (Figure 2.21). Looking to the future, the United Nations predict that, if fertility and mortality decline at a standard rate, then that population will stabilize at 14.2 billion at AD 2100 (high variant), while the low variant predictions (assuming rapid fertility decline and standard mortality decline) predict stabilization around AD 2060 at 8 billion.

The fact that the world is in a demographic transition means exactly that; in most communities there are some people who, sufficiently desperate to control their fertility, will resort to abortion, while there are others who adhere to traditional ways and continue to want large families of four to eight children. Fertility is lower in urban areas where incomes are high, where education is prevalent, where the status of women is high and where women go out to work. However, these are correlates of fertility, not causes. Fertility declines only when people abstain from sex, use contraceptives effectively or have abortions.

In every developing country for which data are available, there is a measurable unmet need for family planning, and people's achieved family sizes exceed their desires. This is not to say that everyone wants to adopt contraceptive methods immediately, but it should direct programming towards increasing the availability of safe, effective and inexpensive methods of contraception and abortion. In broad terms, particularly where government and private medical services are few and far between and overburdened with aspects of curative medicine, this means making oral contraceptives, injectables and condoms available through simple channels; this usually involves their subsidized sale through existing commercial outlets, drawing the doctors back to the provision of voluntary surgical contraception, and dealing with the public health issues associated with abortion.

The twenty-first century

The world has within its grasp a remarkable opportunity. A great deal has been learned about family planning in the first half of the demographic transition: it is a simple, cheap, wanted set of choices that are well understood and that give predictable results. Use has been held back by shortage of resources, restrictive medical practices, confused public policies and general lack of realism. The challenge before the world is to learn from past experience and accomplish the second half of the demographic transition more rapidly. The rate of global population growth has fallen marginally, but absolute numbers continue to rise. By chance, the annual growth in global population is approximately in step with the calendar year: 95 million more births than deaths in 1995, 96 million in 1996 and so on until the end of the decade. More babies will be born in the current decade than in any 10 years in human history. All other considerations apart, unless there is a rapid and marked improvement in contraceptive services, it is possible that more women will die from childbirth and abortion in the last 10 years of this century than in any other decade in the twentieth century. This would be a terrible way to exit our tormented century.

As a result of yesterday's population explosion, there will be one-third more women of fertile age in the year 2000 than there were in 1990. If contraceptive prevalence continues to rise and more women are to be served, then, as a rule of thumb, it may well be possible to double the number of contraceptive users in the present decade.

Some time between now and the year 2010, a year will dawn when there will be fewer babies born than in the year before. The date of this inflexion in the growth of the human population will largely predict the final level of the population of the world. Currently, the United Nations is estimating, at a minimum, a doubling of global population. If family planning continues to receive the low priority it has been given by the international community in the 1980s, then the level of population could well triple. If all unintended pregnancies could be prevented immediately, then the population could stabilize around seven billion.

Affluent Westerners consume much more of the world's resources and pollute much more of its environment than Third World rice farmers or the under-employed or unemployed of Third World urban slums (Figure 2.22). Developmental assistance and political systems are predicated, however, on the principle that poor people will get richer.

Human numbers are already challenging the ability of the biosphere to accommodate the human race. Global grain reserves are getting less, the environment is changing, global warming may have begun, the holes in the ozone layer are enlarging, tropical forests are disappearing, the Sahara is spreading, large areas of the ocean are polluted, and fish yields are falling in many places. Even if these problems can be overcome, finding the capital and job opportunities to employ ever-increasing numbers of young people is an almost impossible challenge.

Some time in the next 100 years the world has to complete the transition from the present energy-intensive industrial societies and intensive agriculture, to a biologically sustainable set of systems. We must move from an economy dependent on fossil fuels and other non-renewable resources to a biologically sustainable economy where we take no more from the environment than living processes can renew, and put no more back into the environment as pollution than the living processes can absorb. This most challenging of transitions must be accomplished while the world also attempts to lift increasingly large numbers of people out of abysmal poverty to some semblance of dignity and freedom from poverty. It may well prove the most technically difficult task the human race has faced. Science can solve many problems and Cassandras have been proved wrong in the past. But as we press at the finite limits of the planet we must remind ourselves that *every* problem must be overcome or irreversible damage will be done at least to parts of our environment.

The final stable population of the world will be a key factor determining success or failure in this ultimate test of political, technical and economic systems. A world of 10 billion people, even given goodwill and luck – which are not always abundantly available – will find it difficult to adjust to twice its present population, particularly as many of these people will be consuming much more than they do at present. A world with three times as many people might well fail to make the adjustment.

The sight of a few tens or hundreds of thousands of people dying of starvation in the horn of Africa or swept into the sea by cyclones in Bangladesh is deeply disturbing. A world where, in order to balance human numbers, a million people might die every 4 days is an unthinkable horror.

People want smaller families, family planning is well understood and cheap to make available. Our children and grandchildren will never forgive today's leaders if we do not take the opportunity for making family planning universally available in the 1990s. The costs would be trivial: the cost of inaction immeasurable (Figure 2.23).

In parts of Europe (e.g. Germany and Italy) the average family size has fallen below two children – that is, the population is imploding. In the developing world, in every country that has been surveyed, women want fewer children than they are having, and wherever there are data available, the proportion of women not wanting any more children has risen in the last 10 years.

There is little or no evidence that Americans want fewer or smaller cars, Indians fewer refrigerators, Scandinavians fewer flights to winter holidays in the sun; or that any of a million other demands for energy and raw materials, or the production of greenhouse gases or ozone-destroying chemicals will decline quickly. People all over the planet want smaller families; failure to respond to that need not only condemns millions of women to suffer the misery of unintended pregnancy – and even death from abortion – but it may well prove the deciding factor in the long-term survival of the fragile ecosystem that is the only home the human family has known or will ever know.

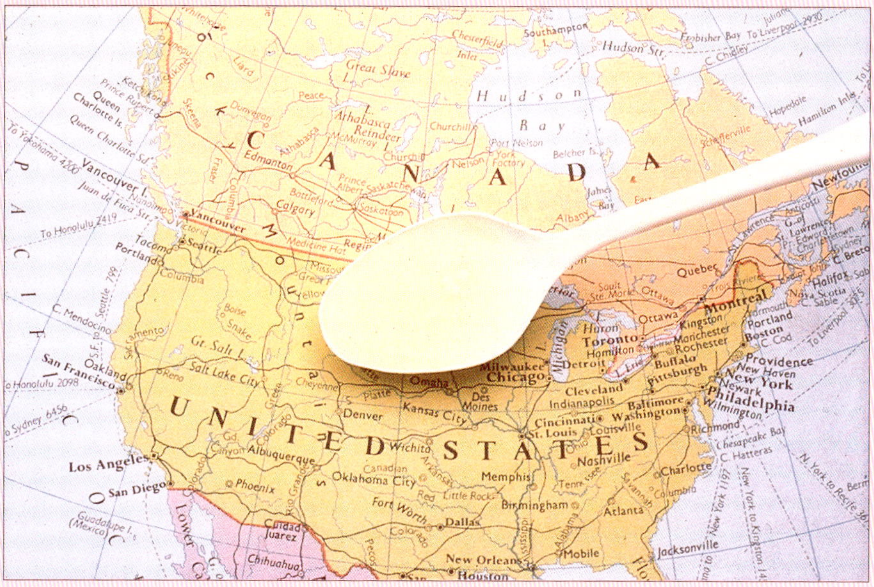

Figure 2.1 A single human ejaculate contained in this teaspoon represents more potential human beings than presently inhabit a large portion of North America. (Reproduced with kind permission from John Guillebaud)

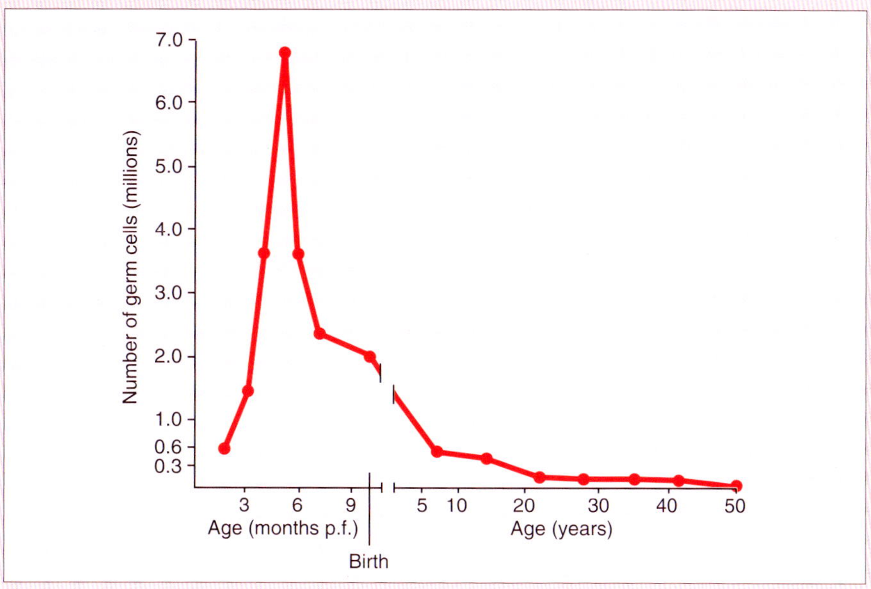

Figure 2.2 Numbers of germ cells in human ovaries (paired) from 2 months primordial follicles (p.f.) to menopausal age. (Adapted from Baker, T. G. (1963). *Proc. R. Soc. London*, **158**, 417)

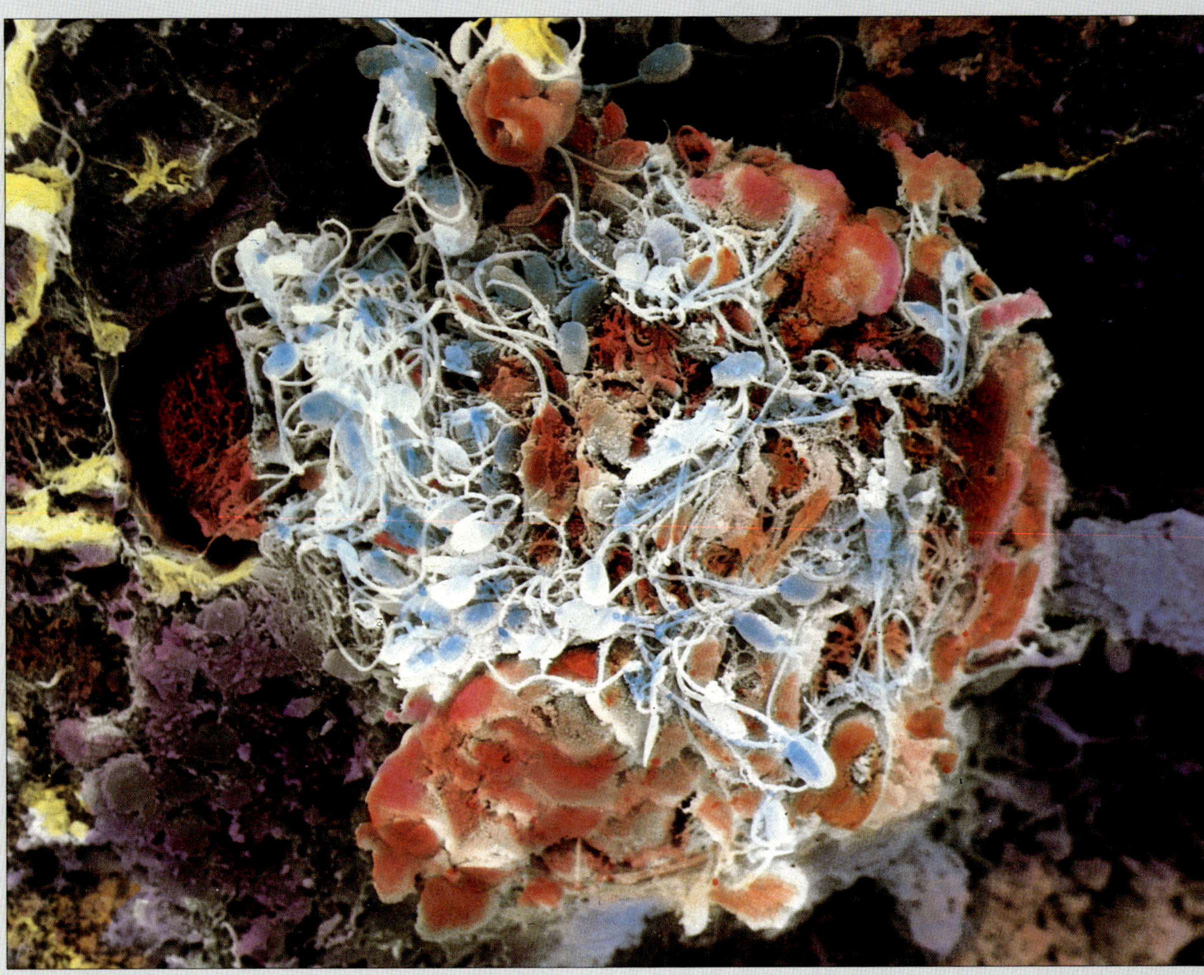

Figure 2.3 Fertilization: false-color scanning electron micrograph of a human egg almost surrounded by spermatozoa (blue). At the beginning of their trip in the vagina, the spermatozoa number about 300 million. The encounter between the egg and the few hundred surviving spermatozoa occurs in the ampullary region of the Fallopian tube. Only one spermatozoon may fertilize the egg and to do this it must penetrate a thick layer of follicular cells (pink) and the inner membrane known as the zona pellucida (not visible here). (Source, Professor P. Motta, University of 'La Sapienza', Rome)

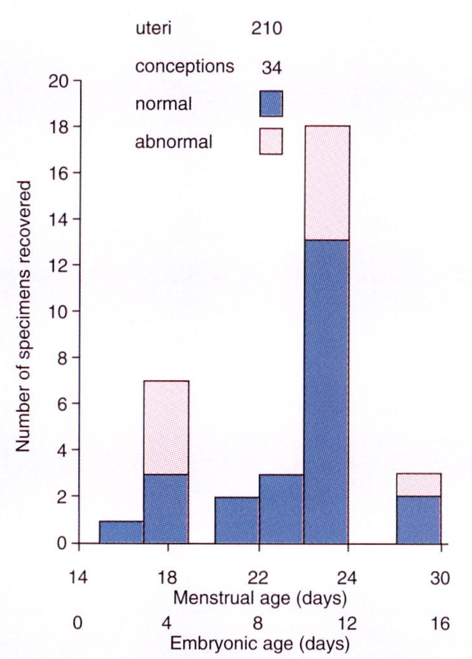

Figure 2.4 Embryonic abnormalities (thought to be incompatible with continuation of the pregnancy) detected prior to and shortly after the first missed period

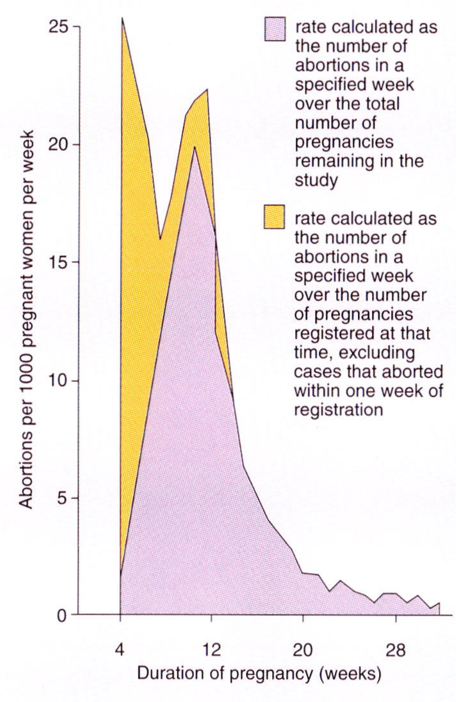

Figure 2.5 Spontaneous abortions by duration of pregnancy

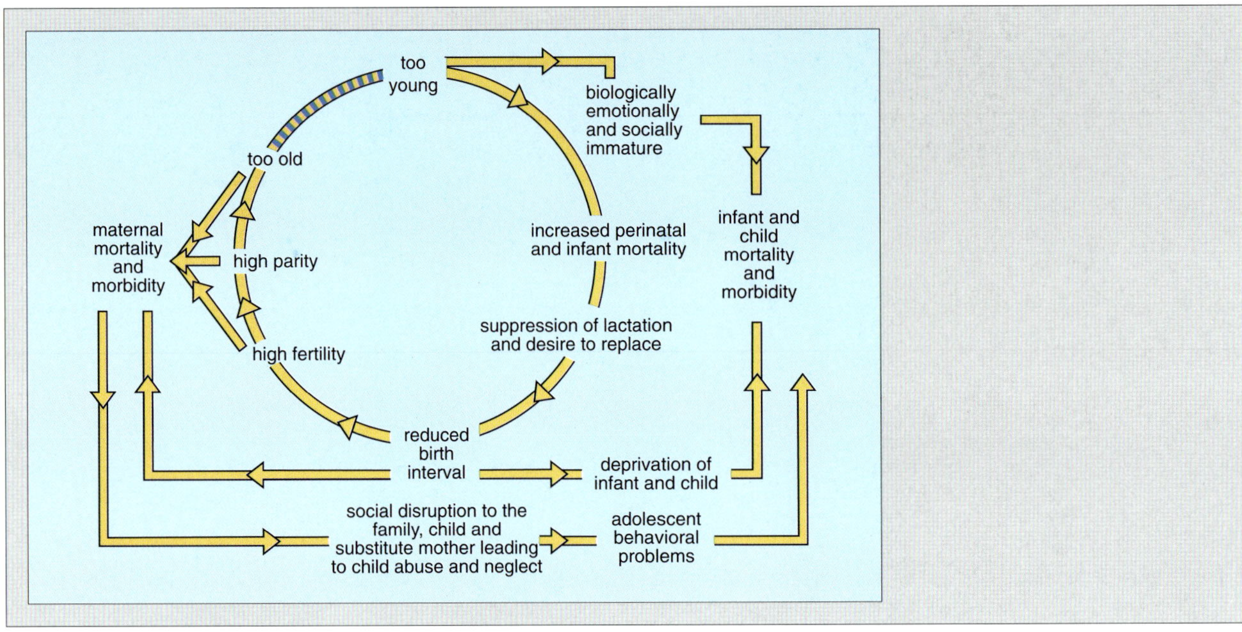

Figure 2.6 'Mothers too young, too old, too frequent, too many'; this scheme shows how these factors interact to increase the risk of maternal and infant mortality and morbidity

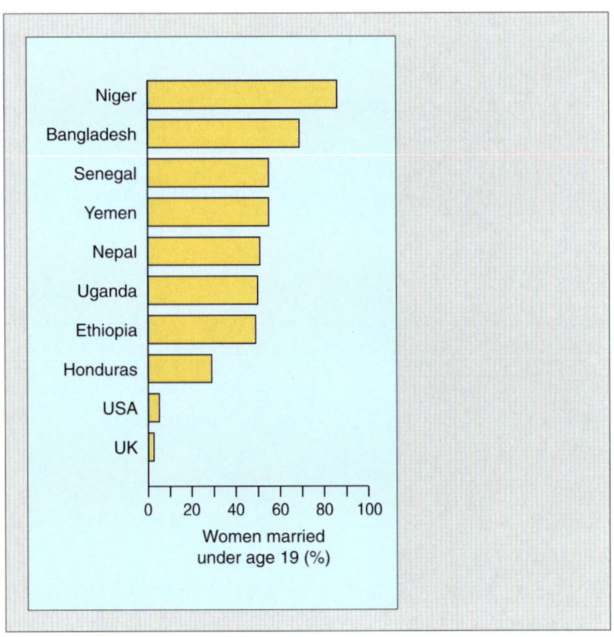

Figure 2.7 Percentage of women married in different countries/continents by age 19 years. (Source, United Nations Nuptuality Chart, 1991)

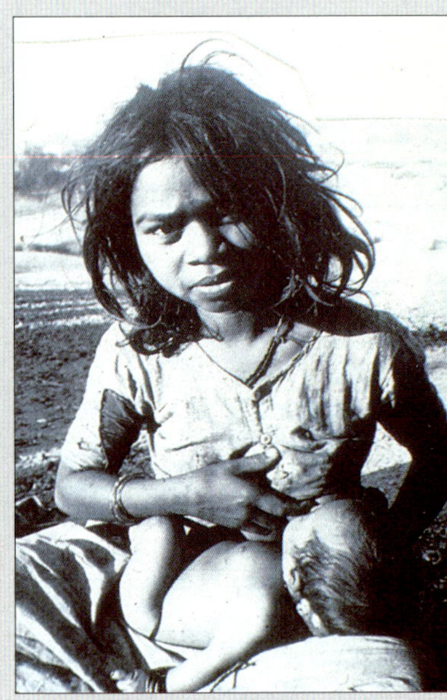

Figure 2.8 Malnourished 12-year-old mother and child. (Source, United Nations Population Fund)

Age (years)	Africa	Asia and Oceania	Latin America and the Caribbean
By 15 years	6%	4%	3%
By 18 years	31%	19%	21%
By 20 years	57%	41%	36%

Figure 2.9 Proportion of women giving birth by age 15, 18 or 20 years among all women aged 20–24, by region (various sources and dates)

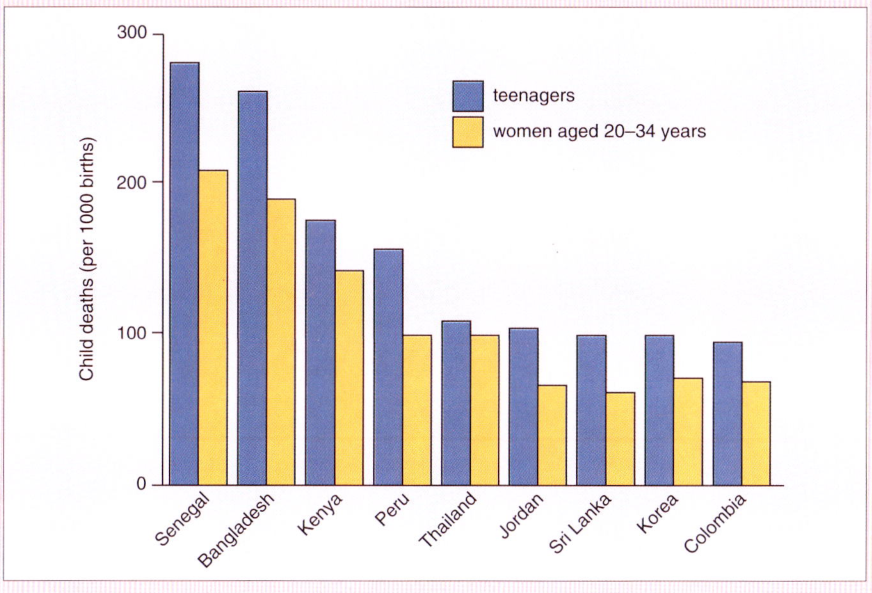

Figure 2.10 Infant mortality by age of mother: selected World Fertility Survey countries. (Adapted from Acsadi, G. T. F. and Johnson-Acsadi, G. (1985). *Family Planning and the Well-being of Women and Children*. (London: International Planned Parenthood Federation))

Country	*Births to women over 35(%)*
Nigeria	15
Senegal	17
Mexico	13
Bangladesh	25
Philippines	16
Sri Lanka	11
USA	21

Figure 2.11 Percentage of all births to women over 35 years of age (mid 1980s)

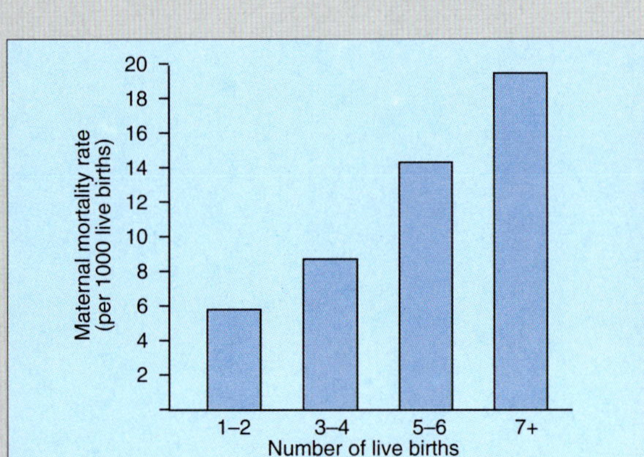

Figure 2.12 Maternal mortality rate by number of live births showing that maternal mortality increases with parity (mid 1980s)

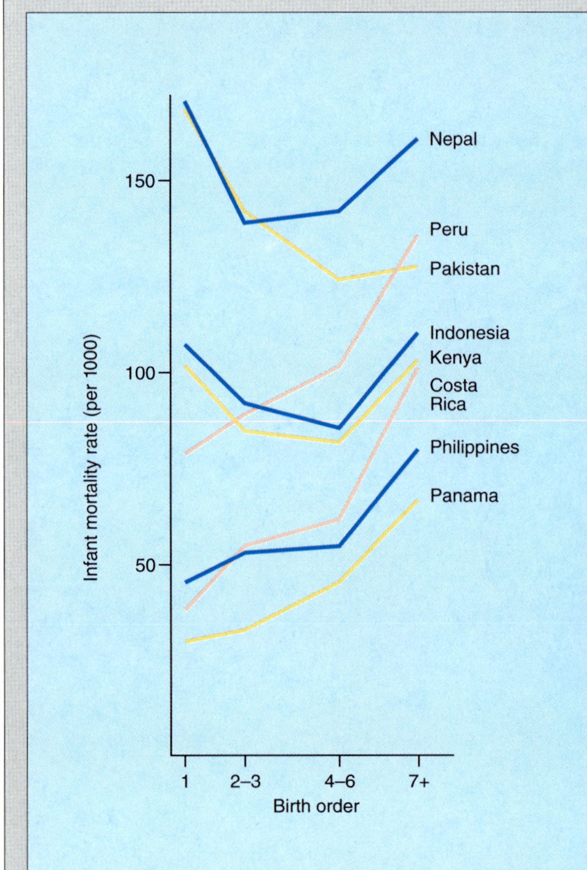

Figure 2.13 Infant mortality by birth order: selected World Fertility Survey countries. (Adapted from Acsadi, G. T. F. and Johnson-Acsadi, G. (1985). *Family Planning and the Well-being of Women and Children*. (London: IPPF))

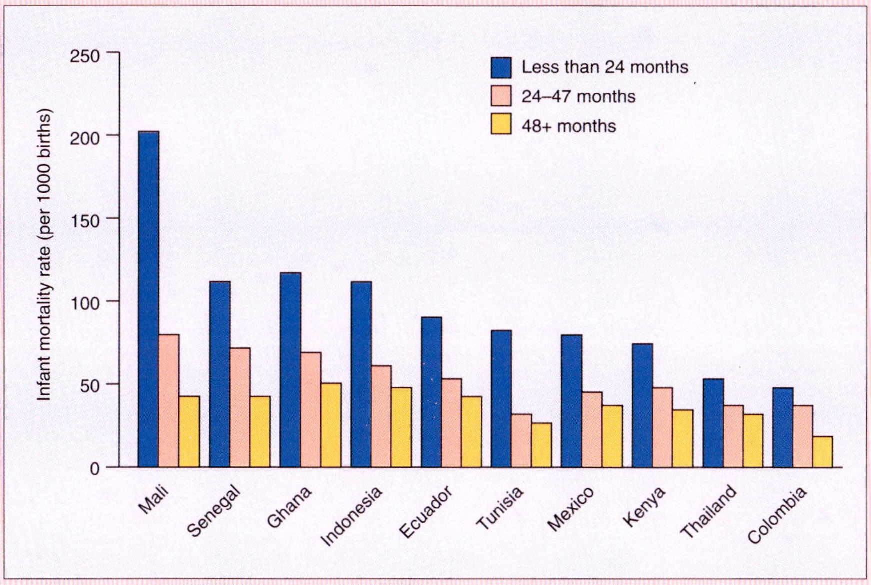

Figure 2.14 Birth spacing reduces infant deaths

Birth interval (months before index child)	Mean Mill Hill vocabulary scores	Mean Raven's Progressive Matrices scores	Mean heights (cm)	Mean weights (kg)	Teachers' assessments	
					>Average (%)	<Average (%)
<12	17.0	23.0	128.2	23.7	8.8	64.0
13–18	18.6	25.0	129.5	24.9	14.7	28.0
19–24	20.6	27.7	130.5	25.5	35.3	8.0
>24	20.9	28.2	131.7	26.3	41.2	0.0

Figure 2.15 Birth interval, measures of intelligence and growth among 560 9-year-old children in Singapore. Results were independent of family size. (Adapted from Martin, C. E. (1978). *J. Trop. Paediatr.*, **25**, 45–76)

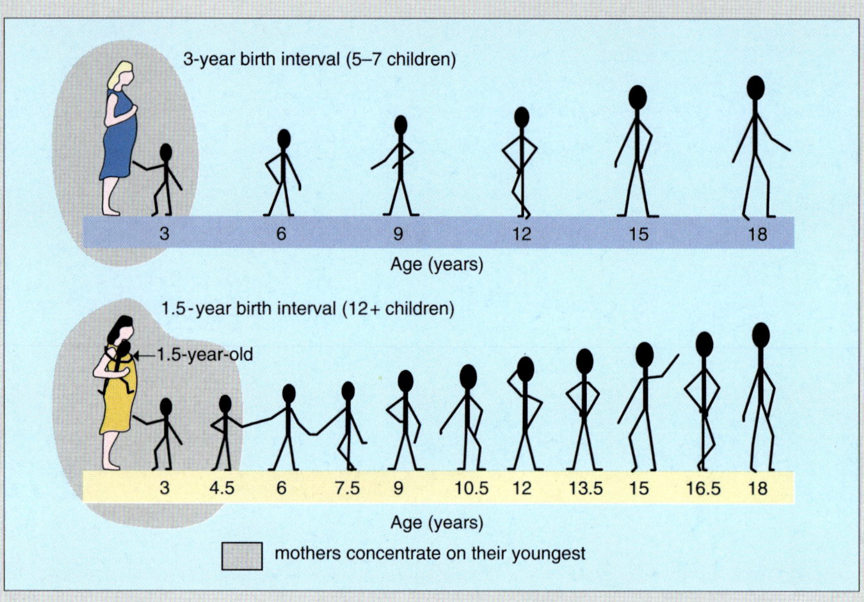

Figure 2.16 Diagrammatic representation of 'traditional' and 'modern' families, demonstrating differences in the amount of attention received by each child. With a 3-year birth interval (5–7 children), when the mother is 6-months pregnant, she has given her youngest 33 months' attention, which has to be shared with one other child. With a 1.5-year birth interval, when the mother is 6-months pregnant, she has given her youngest only 15 months' attention and this has to be shared with two other very young children

Area	*Estimated annual maternal deaths*	*Maternal deaths per 100 000 live births*	*Lifetime risk of dying from pregnancy - related causes*
All developing countries	505 000	420	1 in 57
South Asia	224 000	572	1 in 38
Africa	169 000	640	1 in 25
Latin America	25 000	270	1 in 90
East Asia	30 000	55	1 in 870
All developed countries	4000	26	1 in 1750
North America	1000	12	1 in 4006
Europe	1000	23	1 in 2288
World	509 000	370	1 in 73

Figure 2.17 Maternal death statistics. (Source, World Health Organization, 1992)

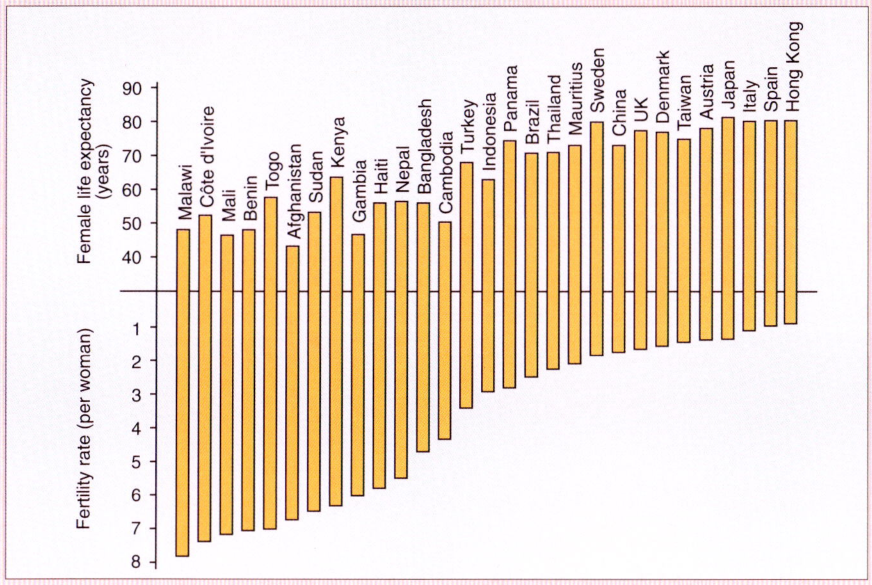

Figure 2.18 Relationship between fertility rates and female life expectancy. (Data obtained from Population Reference Bureau Inc. (1980) in collaboration with UNICEF, *World's Women Data Sheet*, Washington, DC)

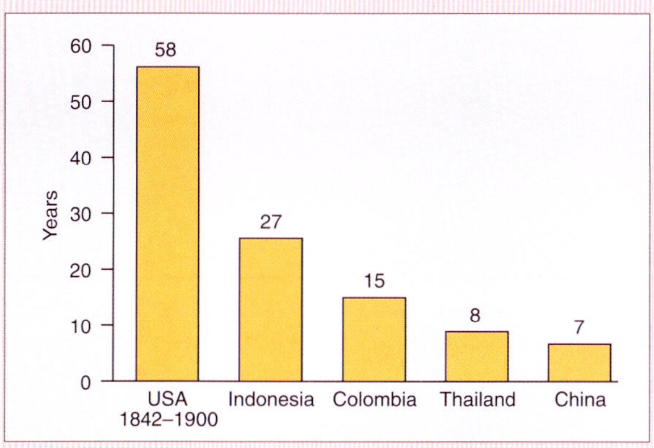

Figure 2.19 Fertility trends in selected countries (expressed as the number of years it took for family size to fall from 6.0 to 3.5). (Adapted from: *The State of World Population, 1991*. (New York: United Nations Population Fund))

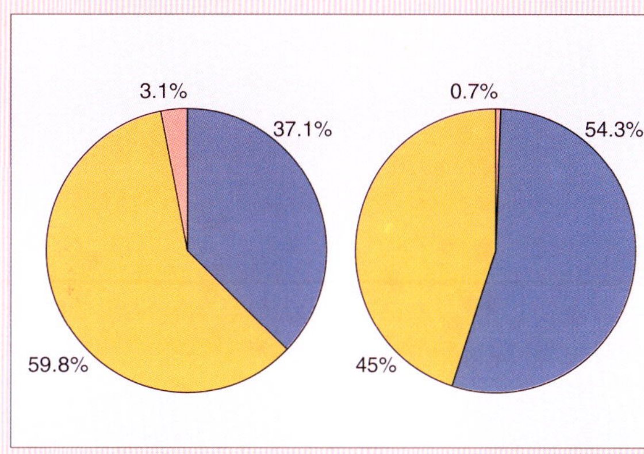

Figure 2.20 The percentage of Protestants, Catholics, and other religious groups in The Canton and city of Basle, 1960 (left), and the percentage of women from these populations having abortions ($n = 320$)(right). Protestant, yellow; Catholic, blue; other religious groups, pink

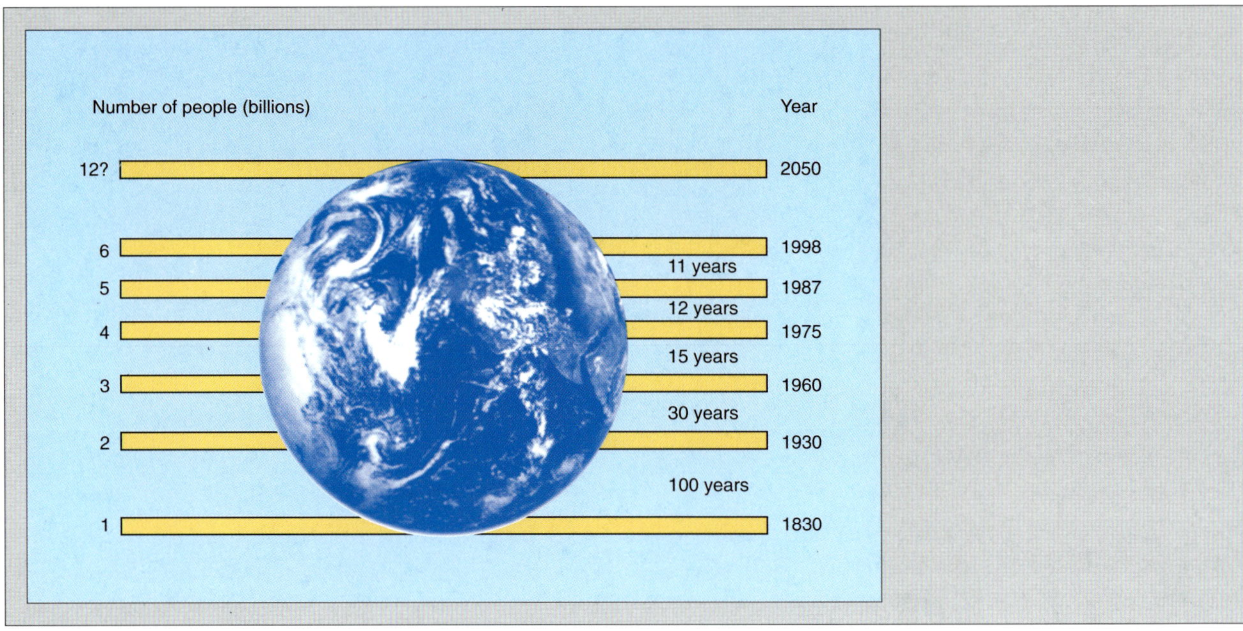

Figure 2.21 The United Nations prediction. The pattern of population increase up to 2050, and the number of years required to add one billion more people

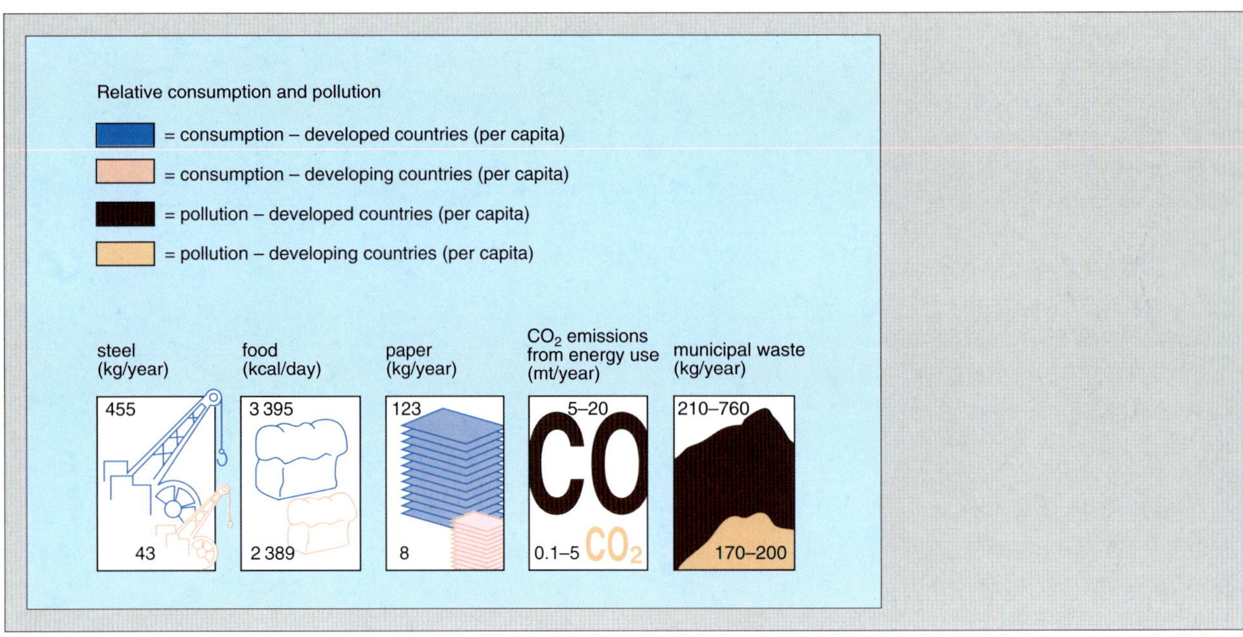

Figure 2.22 Relative consumption and pollution

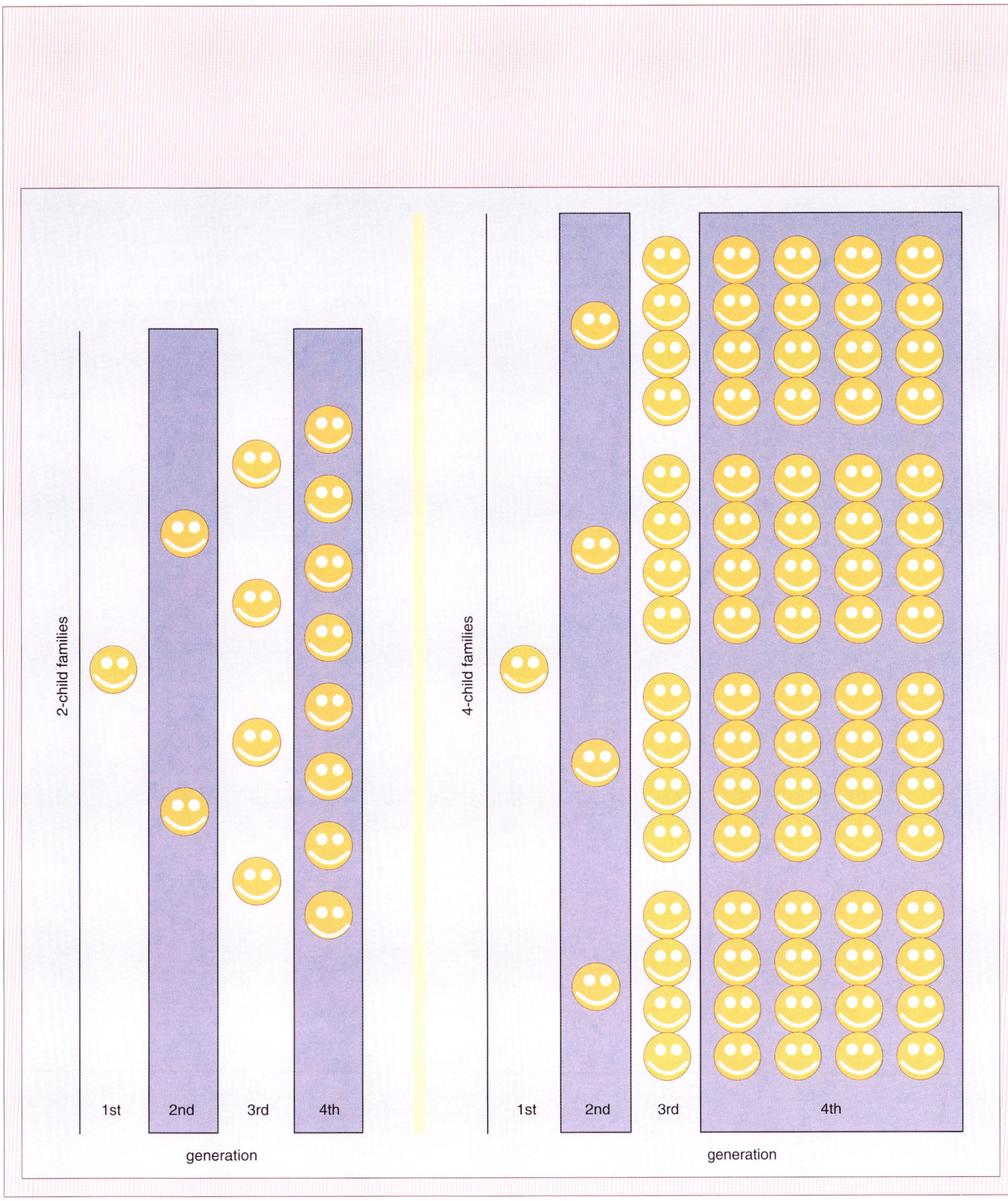

Figure 2.23 Bigger families, faster population growth. Four generations of 2- and 4-child families

3

History of family planning

The history of family planning is the history of conflict between the majority of the community, who are often vividly aware of the socioeconomic needs to restrain fertility, and social elites, who, although they are the first to restrict the size of their own families, tend to maintain the political, legal and ecclesiastical status quo. Conservative attitudes have influenced the rate at which various technologies affecting human fertility have been developed and have diffused throughout society. For example, there were no political, legal or theological comments on the introduction of either wet nursing in the sixteenth and seventeenth centuries or artificial milk formulae in the late nineteenth and twentieth centuries but, by contrast, a great deal of controversy has surrounded the availability of contraceptives and the choices of voluntary surgical contraception and abortion.

The use of coitus interruptus to control fertility is referred to in the Bible and simple barrier methods of contraception are known from ancient Egypt. The history of modern family planning began in the early nineteenth century with the writings of Francis Place, Robert Dale Owen, and John Stuart Mill, in Britain, along with Charles Knowlton in the United States. Society tends to be conservative in most matters of reproduction and it is significant that these early leaders were free thinkers, who rejected contemporary religion.

The Christian rejection of birth control reached its most forceful expression in the writings of Saint Augustine and Saint Thomas Aquinas (1225–74). Augustine argued that original sin was an entity transmitted in the semen, rather like a latter day AIDS virus. In the Bible (*Genesis* 38: 9), Onan 'when he went into his (dead) brother's wife . . . he emitted on the ground, lest he should give an heir to his brother. And the thing which he did displeased the Lord: wherefore he slew him.' Theologians are divided as to whether Onan's sin was to practise coitus interruptus or to disobey his father and not raise children by his dead brother's wife. Be that as it may, Augustine interpreted all forms of contraception as anathema. For a millennium and a half the Catholic and later the Protestant Churches taught that contraception was a sin, in some cases worse than adultery or abortion.

The conflict between orthodox religion and family planning grew during the nineteenth century and has continued to this day. In 1877, Charles Bradlaugh and Annie Besant republished Charles Knowlton's book the *Fruits of Philosophy* (1832). Knowlton had described coitus interruptus, albeit in coy terms; on republication Bradlaugh and Besant were tried and convicted under the Obscene Publications Act, but subsequently acquitted on a technicality. The publicity associated with the trial put contraception 'onto the breakfast tables' of the English middle classes and from 1877 onwards the birth rate in Britain began to decline. In 1873 the United States went in the opposite direction when Anthony Comstock persuaded Congress that anything to do with contraception was an obscenity and that birth control information should not be distributed through the postal system.

In Britain the opposition to family planning was less extreme than in the USA, but almost as destructive; by 1910 15% of English couples had used contraception at some time during their marriage and by 1935–39, two-thirds. But religious teaching remained at variance with the conscience of the flock until the 1920 Lambeth Conference when the Anglican Church cautiously accepted family planning. Catholic teaching continues to reject family planning and in 1968 Pope Paul issued the encyclical *Humanae Vitae*, excluding all methods of contraception except for periodic abstinence. Paradoxically, this was one method which Saint Augustine had specifically and explicitly condemned. In 1993, *Veritatis Splendor* reiterated the well-known teachings of the Roman Catholic Church on contraception.

Margaret Sanger (Figure 3.1) was a public health nurse practicing in New York. One of the women she cared for, Sadie Sachs, was recovering from an illegal abortion. Mrs Sanger asked the doctor how Mrs Sachs might prevent further pregnancies and he flippantly replied that Sadie's husband should 'sleep on the roof'. When Sadie had a second abortion and died, Margaret Sanger was propelled into a life-long crusade for family planning. She published a million copies of her *Family Limitation*. She visited Europe to learn about Mensinga's diaphragm and opened the first family planning clinic in America in Brooklyn in 1916. Under the Comstock laws she was indicted and imprisoned (Figure 3.2).

Eventually the Comstock laws were interpreted so as to permit qualified medical personnel to give contraceptive advice 'for the cure and prevention of disease'. In 1936, in the celebrated case known as 'The United States vs. One Package', Mr Justice Hand further modified the Comstock Acts so as to permit 'the importation, sale or carriage by mail of things that might intelligently be employed by conscientious and competent physicians for the purpose of saving life or promoting the wellbeing of their patients'. The Comstock Acts themselves, however, were not finally struck down until the Supreme Court case of Griswald vs. Connecticut in 1965. These legal precedents made doctors into the fig leaves which society required to make contraception respectable, and they are an important reason why some aspects of family planning have become an over-medicalized set of procedures.

FERTILITY CONTROL A HISTORY OF CONFLICT

Although fertility control, as noted, has had an important impact on the health of women and children, it is not a therapy prescribed to control diseases but a series of choices that informed individuals make. The conflict between private choice and public conservatism, and between science and religion in the field of fertility control has found its expression in the long, acrimonious and still destructive collision between those who would restrict access to family planning or who see it as a series of therapies to be prescribed, and those who see all restrictions as unnecessary and believe that adults have a basic human right to choose from or reject the variety of technologies that now exist to control fertility.

This conflict restrained and confused the medical profession in three overlapping ways. First, for good reasons, the practice of medicine tends to be conservative and this conservatism is transmitted to the rest of society who look to the medical profession for leadership in anything to do with the human body or the health of the family. Second, the perceived need of society to make family planning 'respectable', as so vividly exemplified by Margaret Sanger's history, thrust doctors into a controlling position in family planning even when they were not clinically relevant. Finally, public controversy over family planning retarded scientific investigation.

The US National Institutes of Health, the world's largest funder of medical research, were held back by Congress legislation from working in family planning until 1960. Even in the UK, where greater pragmatism obtained, research into spermicides at Oxford University between the two World Wars led to Dr J. R. Baker being denied the use of the laboratories in the Department of Zoology; Dr Baker was only rescued by Professor Howard Florey, later the Nobel Prize winner for the development of penicillin. In the World Health Assembly, the Vatican State prevented the World Health Organization responding to requests for assistance from developing countries in family planning until 1965.

Be brave and angry

Pioneers of family planning in the West in the nineteenth and early twentieth centuries and more recent leaders in the developing countries have a great deal in common. Despite the efforts of the early campaigners, family planning is still not without obstacles, even in developed countries. In 1990/91, the Irish Family Planning Association was prosecuted in Dublin for selling condoms in the Virgin Music Megastore. The first indictment and appeal were lost and the Association was fined. Efforts have been made in the Irish parliament to introduce more liberal legislation but have not yet succeeded. Poland has, in 1993, reversed previously liberal abortion laws.

In Iran in February 1979, Mrs Farman Farmaian was arrested by young zealots working for Ayattola Khomeini and was almost executed 'for the killing of 5000 infants' – this being the misinterpretation of young religious fundamentalists of visits by 5000 women to a family planning clinic run by Mrs Farmaian.

HISTORY OF CONTRACEPTION

Fertility can be restored to lower levels by the use of contraception, abortion, or a combination of the two. Efforts to control human fertility are as old as written history. Medical papyri from Egypt (Figure 3.3) describe contraceptive suppositories including one based on crocodile dung! In their efforts to prevent or abort pregnancy, women have eaten or drunk various concoctions, roots and plants – many of them poisonous (native Indian women in northern New Brunswick, Canada, brewed dried beaver testicle in a strong alcoholic solution). Contraceptive sponges of different shapes and sizes were dipped in solutions such as soap or vinegar and placed against the cervix. The cervical cap has a history touching on Casanova, that adventuresome lover of the eighteenth century who advocated using a half lemon from which the juice had been extracted. The block pessary gained a bad reputation due to its awkward shape; in 1931 it was considered more an instrument of torture than a prevention of pregnancy (Figure 3.4). The modern intrauterine device (IUD) is only a stone's throw from its origins 3000 years ago; legend has it that smooth pebbles inserted into the uteri of camels prevented them from becoming pregnant during long treks across the desert (Figure 3.5). Today's intrauterine devices owe their designs to the wishbone intracervical pessaries and stem plugs of the early 1900s. Some wishbones were fashioned from 10 and 14 carat gold, and sometimes stem plugs were sutured to the uterus wall to prevent expulsion (Figure 9.1).

Birth control methods have come a long way since the concoctions prescribed in the *Ebers* papyrus, but the perfect contraceptive still remains elusive. Researchers are continually exploring new methods, such as long-acting subdermal implants, contraceptive pellets, female injectables and the much anticipated male oral contraceptive (*see* Chapter 15).

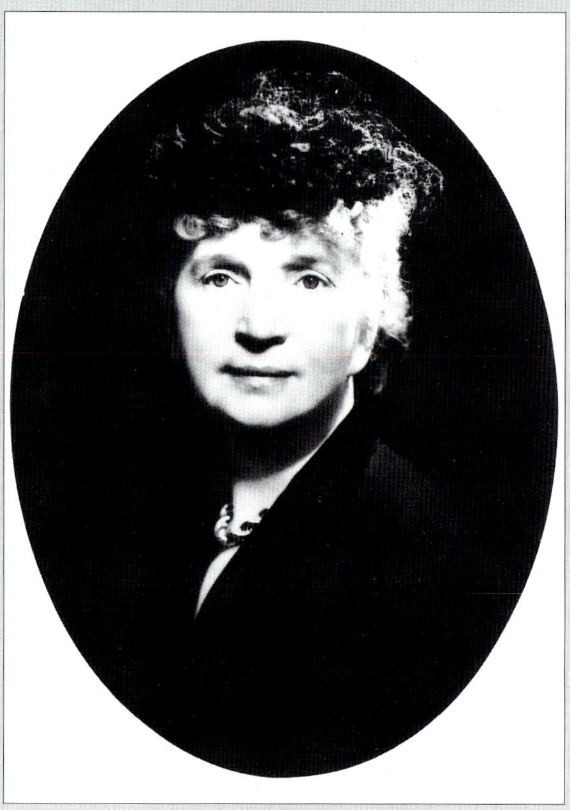

Figure 3.1 Margaret Sanger, an early USA family planning crusader. She opened the first family planning clinic in America in 1916 but was indicted and imprisoned for her efforts

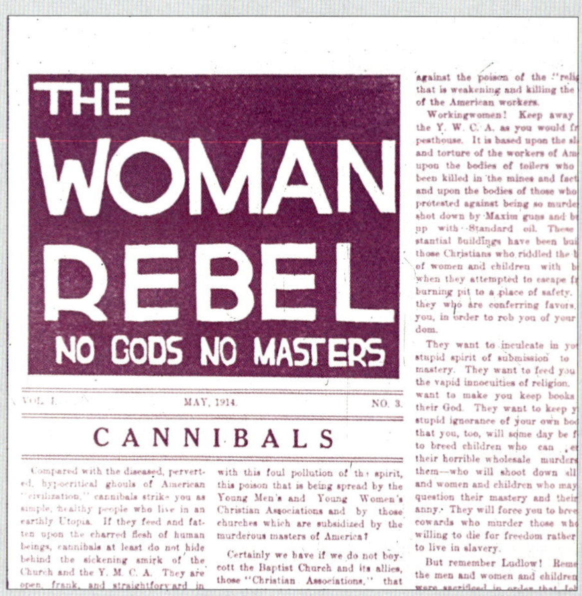

THE WOMAN REBEL

NO GODS NO MASTERS

VOL. I. MAY, 1914. NO. 3.

CANNIBALS

Compared with the diseased, perverted, hypocritical ghouls of American "civilization," cannibals strike you as simple, healthy people who live in an earthly Utopia. If they feed and fatten upon the charred flesh of human beings, cannibals at least do not hide behind the sickening smirk of the Church and the Y. M. C. A. They are open, frank, and straightforward in with this foul pollution of the spirit, this poison that is being spread by the Young Men's and Young Women's Christian Associations and by those churches which are subsidized by the murderous masters of America?

Certainly we have if we do not boycott the Baptist Church and its allies, those "Christian Associations," that against the poison of the "reli that is weakening and killing the of the American workers.

Workingwomen! Keep away the Y. W. C. A. as you would fr pesthouse. It is based upon the sl and torture of the workers of Am upon the bodies of toilers who been killed in the mines and fact and upon the bodies of those who protested against being so murde shot down by Maxim guns and b up with Standard oil. These stantial buildings have been bui those Christians who riddled the b of women and children with b when they attempted to escape fr burning pit to a place of safety. they who are conferring favors you, in order to rob you of your dom.

They want to inculcate in yo stupid spirit of submission to mastery. They want to feed you the vapid innocuities of religion. want to make you keep books their God. They want to keep y stupid ignorance of your own bo that you, too, will some day be f to breed children who can e their horrible wholesale murder them—who will shoot down all and women and children who may question their mastery and their anny. They will force you to bre cowards who murder those wh willing to die for freedom rather to live in slavery.

But remember Ludlow! Reme the men and women and children

Figure 3.2 'The Woman Rebel: No Gods, No Masters'. Margaret Sanger's case as reported in the media

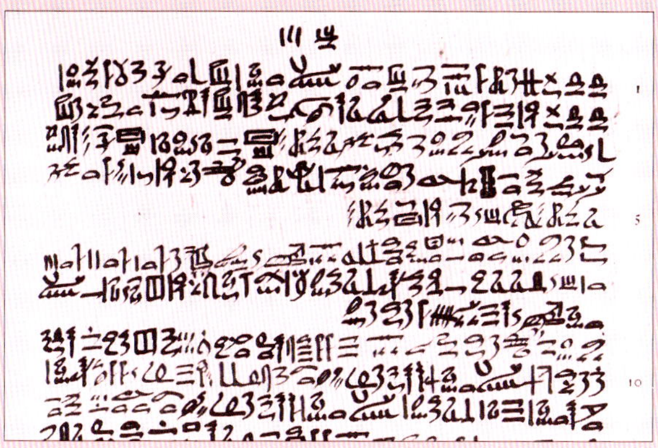

Figure 3.3 The *Ebers* papyrus dates back to 1550 BC; it recommends a medicated tampon designed 'to cause that a woman should cease to conceive for 1, 2, or 3 years'. The ingredients include seedwool moistened with honey, ground acacia and dates. (Courtesy of the IPPF)

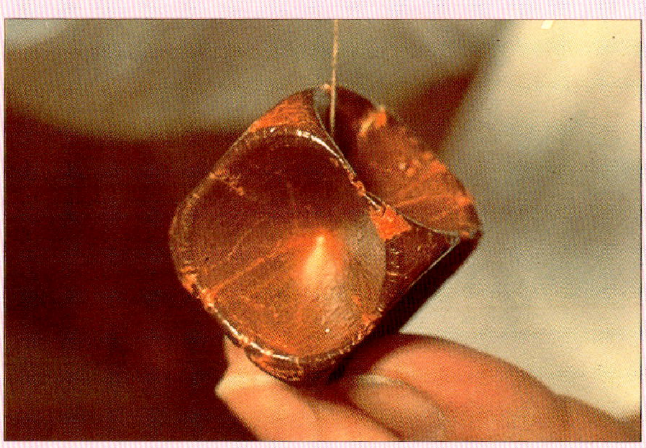

Figure 3.4 One of the most unusual barrier methods was the block pessary which was inserted into the vagina in the hope that one of the concave surfaces would fit over the cervix. It was described as an instrument of torture. (Reproduced with kind permission from Ortho-McNeil Inc., Canada)

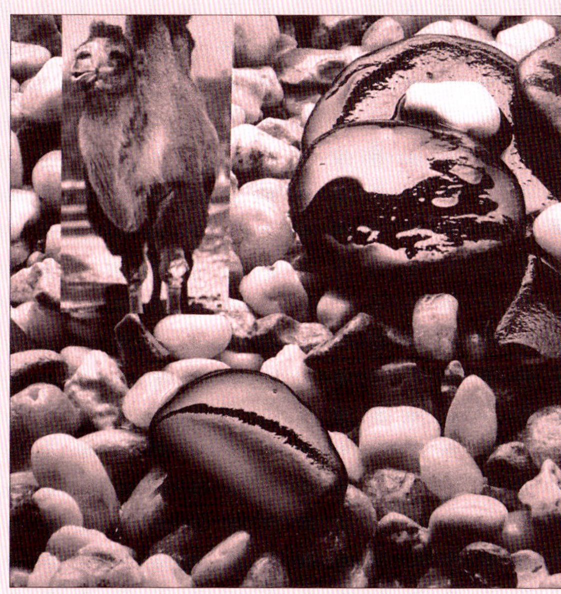

Figure 3.5 The modern intrauterine device (IUD) may have originated from the practice of placing smooth pebbles in the uterus of a camel to prevent it from becoming pregnant during long treks across the desert. (Courtesy of the IPPF)

4

Human sexuality including female reproduction and male physiology

SEX AND REPRODUCTION

It is usual to begin by describing the anatomy and physiology of human reproduction but these attributes can only be understood in a broader context of human sexual behavior.

The human species, like other animals, is judged by evolution according to the number of its offspring that survive to the next generation and reproduce. The male (Figure 4.1) and female anatomies, reproductive physiology and behavior have been tailored over millions of years of evolution to provide for the optimal performance. As a viviparous animal that usually bears one young alive at a time, after a long interval of pregnancy and before an even longer interval of lactation, the anatomy, physiology and behavior of the two sexes are very different: the woman provides a disproportionate share of the energy and time which must be devoted to reproducing the next generation. A woman can only conceive, feed and care for a relatively small number of children in her relatively brief fertile life, while a man, if he is ruthless and competitive, can father a relatively large number of children.

The size of the testicles and the number of sperm produced by men, in relative terms, are less than those among chimpanzees, who are highly promiscuous in their mating, but more than in truly monogamous primates, such as the Marmoset monkey. Men make enough sperm for intercourse a few times a week, rather than perhaps several times a day, as do chimpanzees.

BRAIN AND BEHAVIOR

The primary and largest sex organ in the human species is above the waist – the brain. It has been plausibly argued that every aspect of other systems (the locomotive system, nervous system, etc.) has been driven in evolution by the need to reproduce. The very large brain that characterizes our species, and enables us to read and write books, may have evolved as a result of sexual competition within our own species. After all, some animals with very small brains, such as the dinosaurs, lived on this earth much longer than the human species is likely to survive, and others, such as rats, exploit almost as many different environments as we do. Once an animal evolves a certain proficiency in finding its food, then competition in reproduction comes not from the outside world but from other members of the species and even of the same sex. Possibly our big brains evolved so that we can manipulate one another in the endless competition to secure a mate and to build the bonds between the sexes which are essential to bring up a baby whose brain is so large that it endangers the life of the mother during delivery and who requires continuous close attention for many years during its own development.

The other large apes to whom we are so closely related (human beings and chimpanzees have 98% of their DNA in common) are either polygamous (as is the gorilla) or promiscuous (as are chimpanzees). The males compete with one another for access to the females and, although they may guard the territory from which the females draw their food supply, they play no role in bringing up the next generation.

At some point in relatively recent evolution, the human newborn achieved a threshold size of brain, becoming so totally dependent for so long an interval of time that it was in the biological interest of both sexes to work together to nurture their offspring. In all human societies (although to varying degrees), males accept paternity for their children and make a direct contribution to their upbringing. The key event in the evolution of human sexual behavior, that made the change from a promiscuous primate, like a chimpanzee, to the partially monogamous mating system found in human kind, was the concealment of ovulation in the female.

Human beings are alone among other species in that ovulation in women is not associated with the physical changes seen in other primates (such as the vivid vulval swellings of chimpanzees or baboons), or the behavior changes of estrus seen in other mammals (such as the domestic cat). Men and women can have sexual intercourse on any day of the menstrual cycle, during much of pregnancy, lactation and after the menopause. Two things follow from this unusual form of behavior. First, the male mating strategy has switched from coitus with any available ovulating female to establishing a long-term relationship with one woman – a relationship of love founded on sexual desire and passion. But, a state bordering on perpetual sexual arousal and receptivity, among the adults of an intensely social animal (which we most obviously are) also brings in its wake some secondary problems.

Evolution appears to have built in some additional behaviors to prevent our species falling into sexual chaos: again, if we think of how other animals behave, we are the only species where adults, in all known societies, cover their genitals in public, and all adults in all known societies normally make love in private, commonly after dark and usually isolated from other members of their social group.

Behavior leaves no fossil record and it is impossible to be certain by which specific steps our mating system evolved from our *Australopithicene* ancestors, but concealed ovulation, secret copulation and covering our external genitalia – even totally naked aboriginal tribes in Australia used to stand back to back and talk to one another when adults from different clans met – are unique behavioral strategies that appeared relatively recently in our evolution and are the basis of the human mating system. They are also probably the key to understanding the need for, and the politics of, family planning: most episodes of sexual intercourse are manifestly not for procreation, but to reinforce the bond of sexual love between parents; and yet we are all shy about sex and, just as we cover our external sex organs in public, so we – not unnaturally – find discussion of sex difficult, and often make mistakes in establishing public policies relating to reproduction.

ENDOCRINE CONTROL

Both men and women produce the same set of pituitary and gonadal hormones. In women, libido is also thought to depend on circulating testosterone. However, the pituitary control of follicle stimulating hormone (FSH) and luteinizing hormone (LH) is very different.

The male secondary sexual characteristics and sexual behavior are primarily driven by testosterone, although there is no close correlation between the frequency of intercourse and testosterone levels, and neither has any consistent difference in male physiology been discovered in the case of men who choose a homosexual lifestyle.

Modern civilized living has brought about relatively few changes in the way that males use their reproductive systems – other than an important decline in the age of the onset of puberty. But in women, modern living brings about profound changes, with important life-long consequences.

Many textbooks on medicine look upon the 28-day menstrual cycle as a normal situation for a healthy adult woman. In reality, the reproductive system was evolved to do just that – to reproduce. When healthy women have unprotected intercourse, about one-third of them become pregnant in the first cycle and the majority after three or four cycles. The natural situation is for FSH and LH to control ovulation, and then for FSH and LH produced by the fertilized egg to block the disruption of the endometrium. If conception does not take place, the endometrium is shed; the embryo and fetus have 'highjacked' the female reproductive system (Figure 4.2).

CONCEPTION, PREGNANCY AND DELIVERY

All the eggs that a woman will release are set aside during fetal life. The male produces sperm from puberty to death. Sperm take approximately 120 days to mature. There are large variations in semen volume, sperm number, morphology and motility. Apart from extreme values, the sperm count is not of great value as a predictor of fertility.

The many variations in female reproduction include differences in anatomy, physiology and behavior. Human beings have a single uterine chamber, as opposed to the two horns found in many cattle (and in rare abnormalities in human beings); the cervix is firm and mucus-filled and ejaculation takes place in the vagina, whereas, in horses, the cervix admits the penis and ejaculation takes place in the uterus itself; the vagina is a single passage and not a double tube, as in kangaroos.

The human baby is immature, although not as blind and helpless as some other mammalian species (e.g. cats or bears). The human placenta is hemochorial, unlike say in pigs, where there is less erosion of the maternal and fetal tissues and less chance of severe hemorrhage during delivery as can so tragically affect human delivery.

THE MIRACLE OF LACTATION

'Mother', 'mummy', 'mamma', 'milk', all come from the same linguistic root: we belong to the zoological order Mammalia – and that means we breastfeed our babies.

The human infant depends for its life on its mother's milk. Milk not only nourishes the survival and growth of the child, but the fat content of the milk changes as the child matures and, for example, is adjusted to the needs of the growing brain. Milk is also loaded with antibodies (beginning with the colostrum) and maternal white cells that not only fight infection, but are tailored exactly to cure infections the mother has met in her environment. (The 'piglet in shit' survives because it receives protective antibodies from its mother living in the same insanitary environment.) Milk also contains a factor that assists in the maturation of the baby's gut. Research shows that the protection given, if a mother breastfeeds for the first three months, against intestinal and respiratory infections persists until at least the end of the first year of life. Breastfeeding also reduces a mother's risk of breast cancer later in life.

It is the gonadotropin production from the early embryonic placenta which prevents the onset of the next menstruation; it is the pituitary hormones of the fetus which set the time of delivery. The newborn continues to be in control of the suckling process. The amount of suckling by the baby determines prolactin levels; this is the way by which the infant 'orders its next meal' and suckling is also the key factor in the suppression of ovulation during breastfeeding

(Figure 4.3). As we have seen, in preliterate societies the duration of postpartum lactational amenorrhea is a key factor in the spacing of pregnancies, which in turn is a major factor in determining the risks of pregnancy to the mother and to the newborn infant, or the already existing older sibling.

It is the fact that ovulation is naturally suppressed during pregnancy and breastfeeding which has permitted the development of oral contraceptives which mimic these two processes, albeit somewhat imperfectly. The fact that there is no similar interruption in the male production of sperm is the primary reason why we do not yet have a 'male pill'.

CHANGING PATTERNS OF REPRODUCTION

The time from the birth of one child until the birth of the next is called the birth interval (Figure 4.4). It consists of three parts:

(1) The time taken to conceive;

(2) The duration of pregnancy; and

(3) An interval without ovulation after delivery or abortion.

The pregnancy interval can vary from less than a year to the extremes of a fertile lifetime.

In the absence of contraception, most women fall pregnant within three months of beginning regular intercourse. In a traditional society not using contraceptives but breastfeeding for natural intervals, children are born 3–5 years apart. If breastfeeding is curtailed but not replaced by contraceptives, as in the North American Hutterites (a Protestant religious sect) then the average woman may have nine or ten live births in a life-time.

An induced abortion prevents a birth but if the couple do not use contraceptives the woman may conceive again very rapidly and several abortions can occur in the same interval of time that it takes for a woman to conceive, deliver and breastfeed a baby. Where abortion is combined with contraceptive use, the average time from initiating use until contraceptive failure becomes the largest element of the three components separating two pregnancies and the interval represented by conception and abortion and conception and delivery are more nearly equivalent.

With reduced family size, widespread premarital sexual intercourse (Figures 4.5 and 4.6), and late marriage, life-long patterns of reproduction in the West are now profoundly different from those characterizing earlier ages.

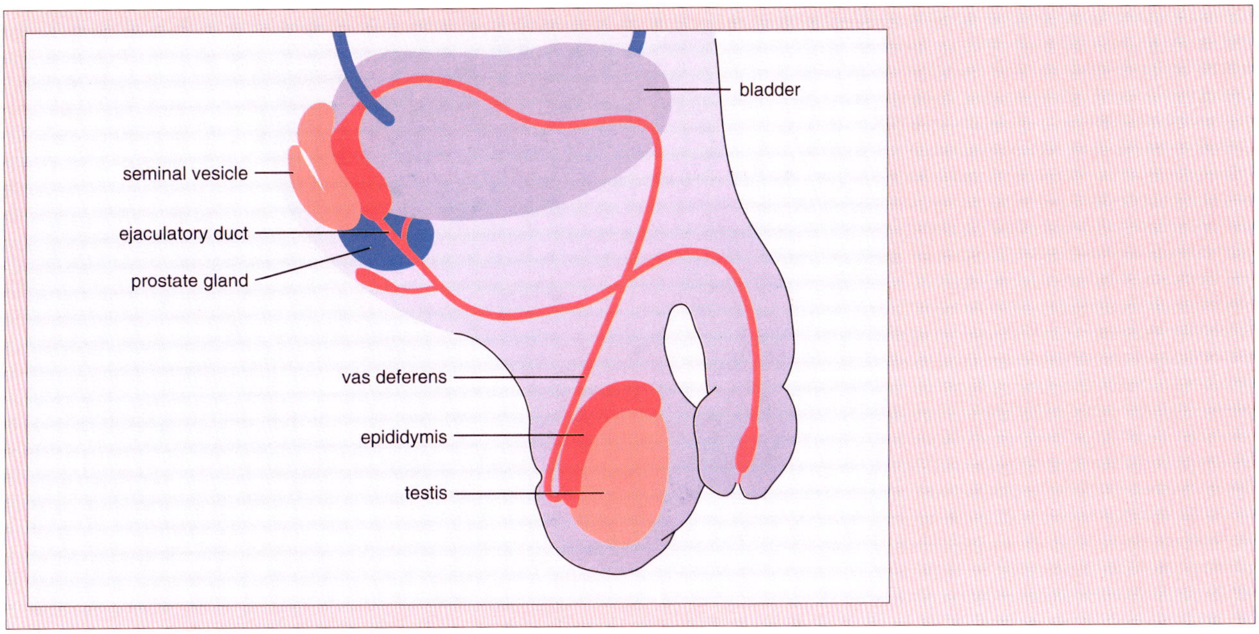

Figure 4.1 Male reproductive anatomy

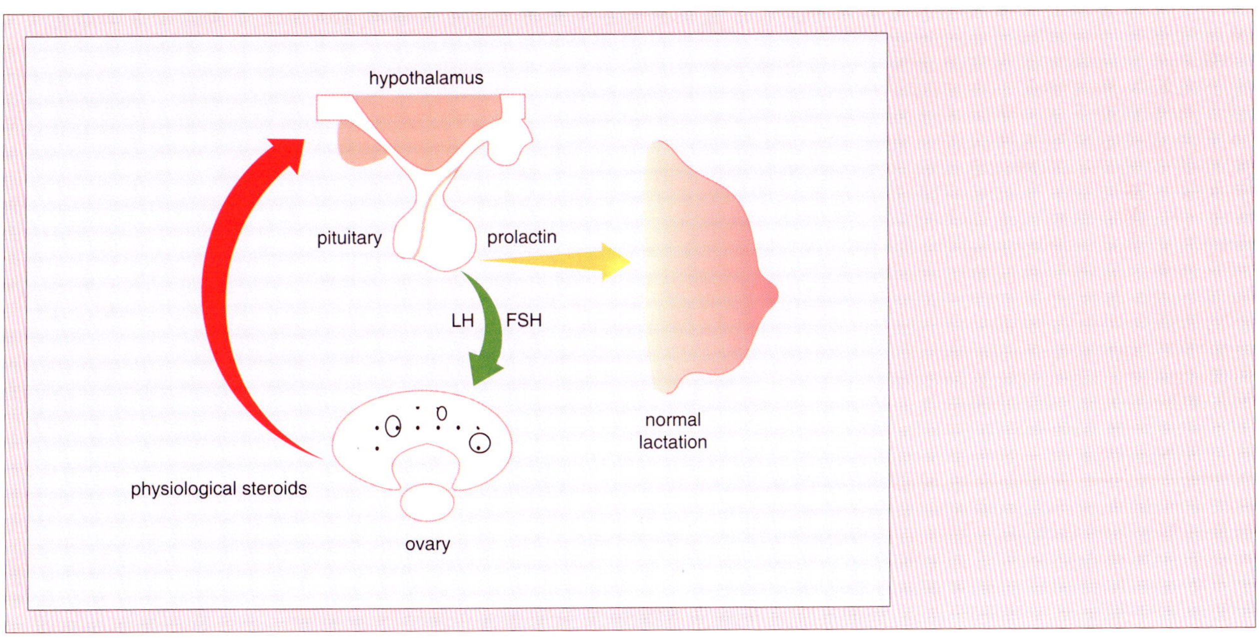

Figure 4.2 Hormonal cycles in the female

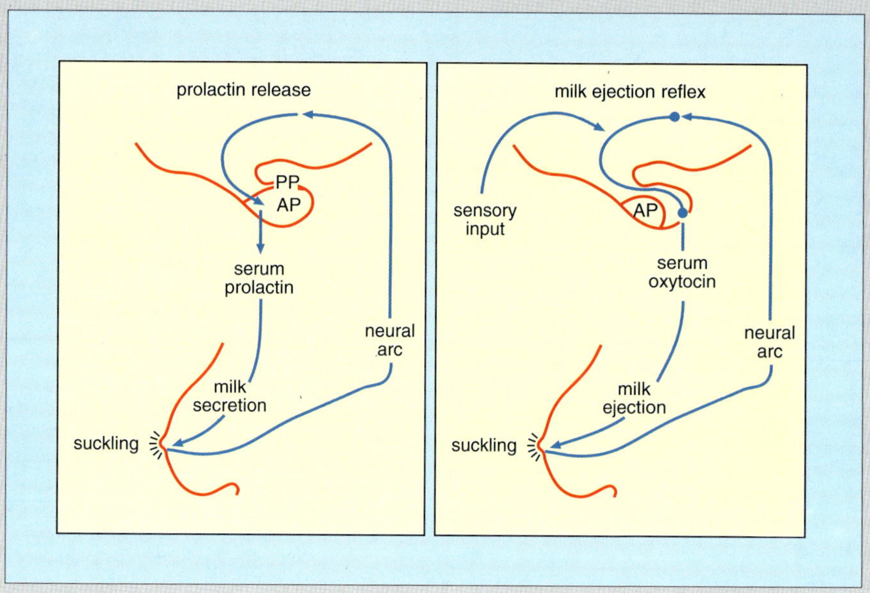

Figure 4.3 Diagrammatic representation of the pathways involved in suckling-induced prolactin and oxytocin release. Both hormones are released in response to nipple stimulation during suckling. The release of these hormones is otherwise independent. Prolactin release does not occur in response to other stimuli associated with nursing while oxytocin release resulting in milk ejection may occur simultaneously or be induced by, for example, the cry of the infant. PP, posterior pituitary; AP, anterior pituitary

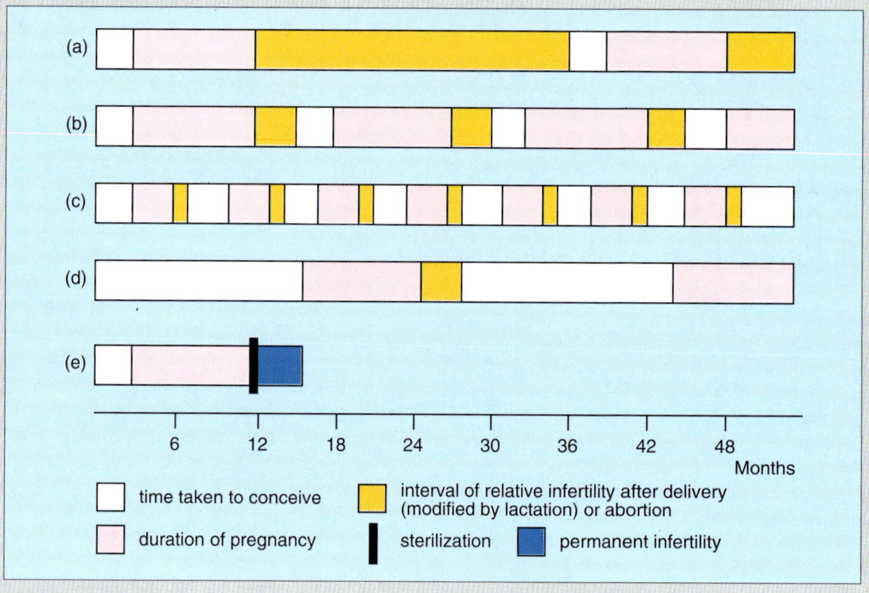

Figure 4.4 Patterns of human reproduction (a) term delivery followed by breastfeeding; (b) term delivery followed by artificial feeding, wet-nursing or stillbirth; (c) spontaneous or induced abortion; (d) use of contraceptives followed by term

Country or territory	*Age range (years)*	*% sexually experienced*	
		Male	*Female*
Australia	by age 20	58	47
Germany	by age 16	35	30
Israel	14–16	42	11
Japan	16–21	15	7
Nigeria	14–19	68	43
Rep. of Korea	12–21	17	4

Figure 4.5 Percentages of adolescents reported to have experienced premarital coitus (selected countries)

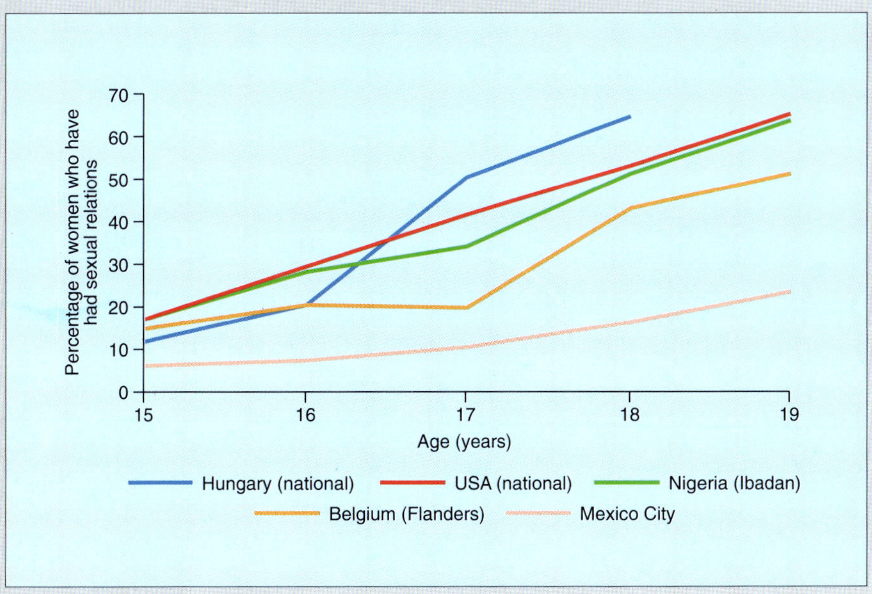

Figure 4.6 Percentage of women who have had sexual relations before marriage

5

Service delivery

Family planning involves three dynamic and interactive elements: fertility regulation methods, the nature of the service delivery system and the perceptions and characteristics of the user (Figure 5.1). Experience shows that a change in a delivery system can be every bit as important in extending family planning choices as the invention of a new method. A new channel of distribution may meet the users' perceptions more closely, as when oral contraceptives are made available to men to give to their wives in a male-dominated society (Figure 5.2) or simply make it more convenient for users to obtain a method (Figure 5.3). The closest and quickest place to obtain contraceptives is often the neighborhood pharmacy, where approximately 50% of the world's couples obtain their temporary family planning supplies (e.g. oral contraceptives, condoms, etc.). In both rich and poor countries most people have neither the time nor the inclination to travel long distances to obtain health care, let alone family planning services (Figure 5.4).

Health personnel have become unusually closely involved in family planning for two reasons: one licit and one accidental. Several methods (e.g. intrauterine devices or vasectomy) necessarily involve medical skills for their safe use. The accidental relationship is more subtle and probably also more important. When family planning is introduced into any community, it is commonly perceived as controversial and even socially disruptive. Doctors, in particular, give family planning an air of respectability. Provider attitudes and availability of different contraceptive methods are linked closely and often remain more important than user perspectives in determining contraceptive availability and use in many countries, for example, hormonal contraception and IUDs are not licenced for contraceptive use in Japan (Figure 5.5).

Medical care, for good reason, is conservative and is necessarily overwhelmed by a diagnostic/therapeutic relationship between the physician and patient. Family planning is profoundly different and health professionals are no more than a 'fertility taxi driver' taking the user to their chosen fertility destination (Figure 5.6).

To further complicate a confusing situation, physicians (e.g. Tamayo in Colombia, Baird in the UK, Guttmacher in the USA, and Yang in Korea) have often been leaders in family planning, motivated by their personal, face-to-face experience of the anguish of unintended pregnancy and the pain of dangerous, exploitive abortions. But, at the same time, medical barriers to access to contraception (Figure 5.7) have evolved into what may be the single most important impediment to the progress of family planning in many parts of the world.

In practice, family planning benefits from the maximum diversity of channels of contraceptive distribution, and almost invariably the consumer will prove better at 'integrating' a variety of contraceptive services than any planner. Not only do people differ in their individual needs, but the same person, or couple, may get their fertility regulation from different sources as they make their life-long fertility journey: a young man may buy condoms from a slot machine, his fiancé may visit a family planning clinic for the pill, but get an intrauterine device from her gynecologist after their first child; she may choose NORPLANT® after their last wanted child, or her husband may go to their family physician for a vasectomy.

Contraceptive advertising is sometimes forbidden by statute law, or industry guidelines. Some developing countries with natural family planning programs still impose import duties on contraceptives.

In developing countries, social marketing (Figures 5.8 and 5.9) may bring condoms and pills into corner shops and kiosks, a community-based distribution service may save vulnerable groups such as teenagers, and private doctors may provide abortions, and the government hospital voluntary surgical contraception. Diversity is the rule of success of programs, and pragmatism the recurrent song of those seeking the maximum impact for their services. Wherever and however the service is provided, respect for the client is paramount. Every client should have a right to information, to access, to choice of method, to safety, to privacy, to confidentiality, to dignity, to comfort, to continuing services and a right to express their opinion (Figure 5.10)

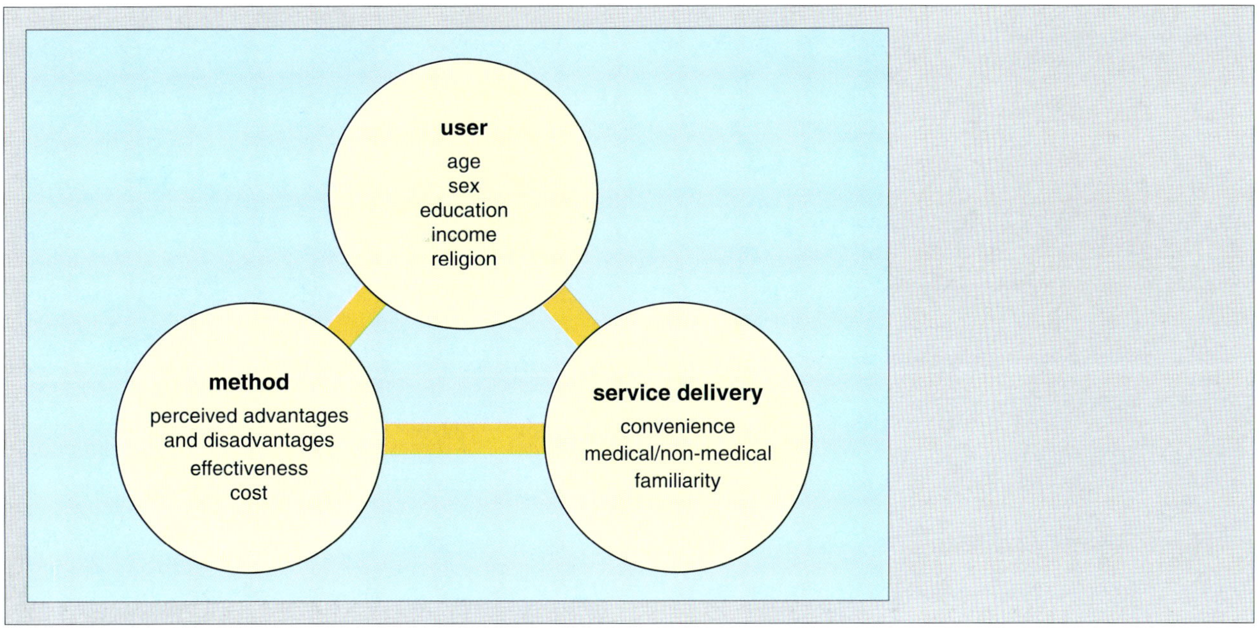

Figure 5.1 Family planning: an interaction between users, methods and channels of delivery

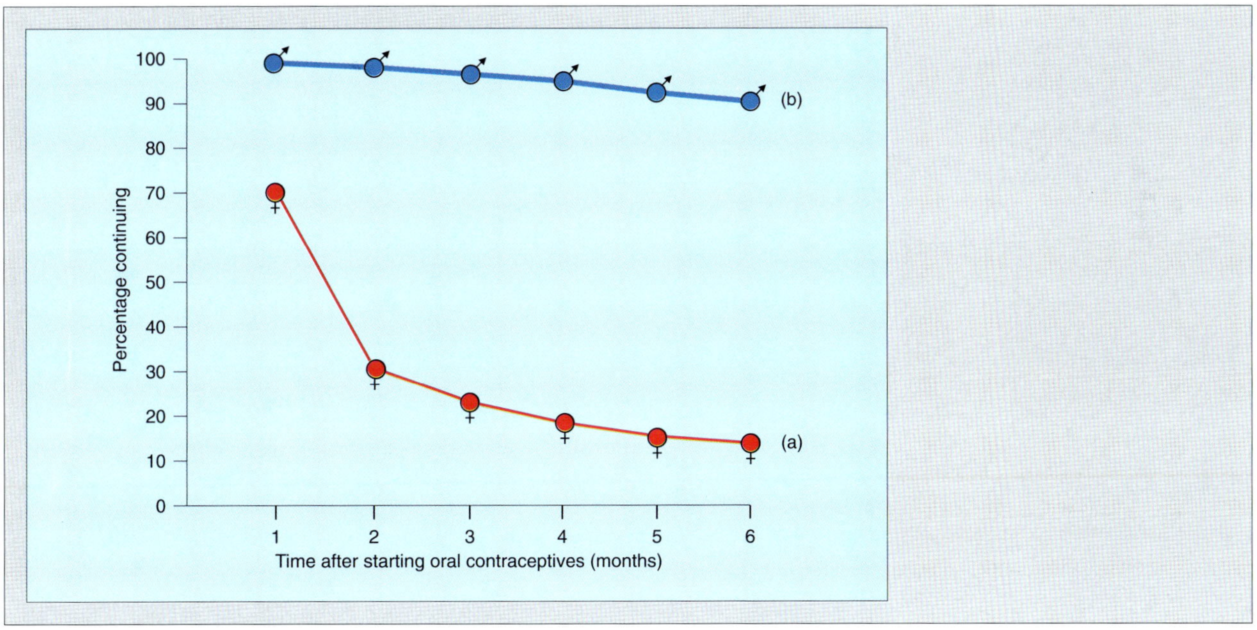

Figure 5.2 Continuation rate for oral contraceptive use in Iran (a) oral contraceptives given by health personnel to women; (b) oral contraceptives given to husbands to pass to their wives

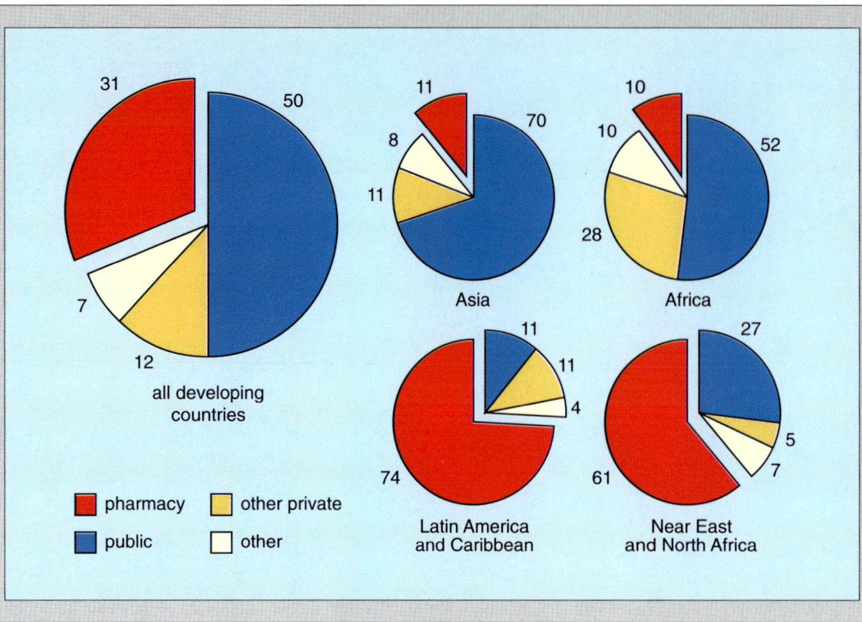

Figure 5.3 Users of condoms, oral contraceptives, injectables or vaginal methods by source of supply (percentages) – estimates for developing areas. (Based on data from Demographic and Health Surveys. Excludes China)

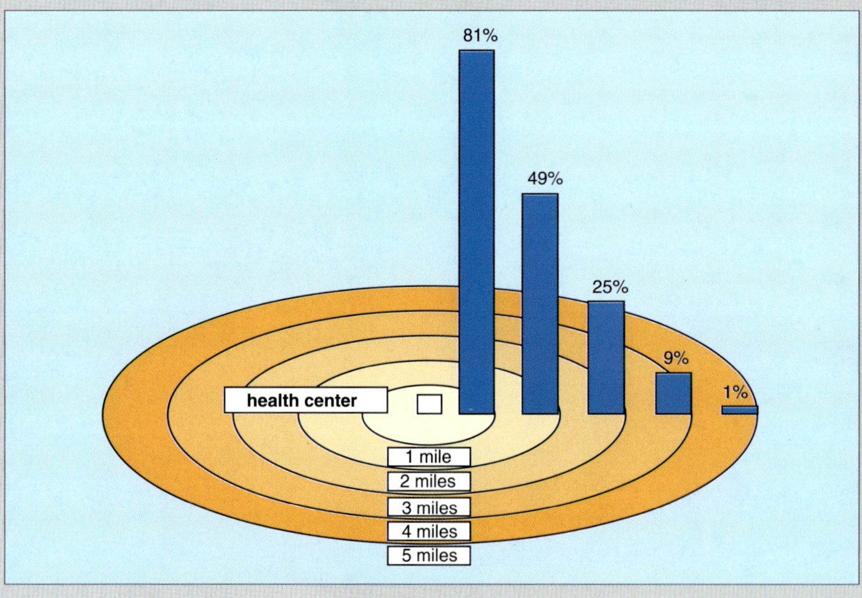

Figure 5.4 Utilization of health services (expressed as a percentage of health center clients) according to the distance traveled by the client

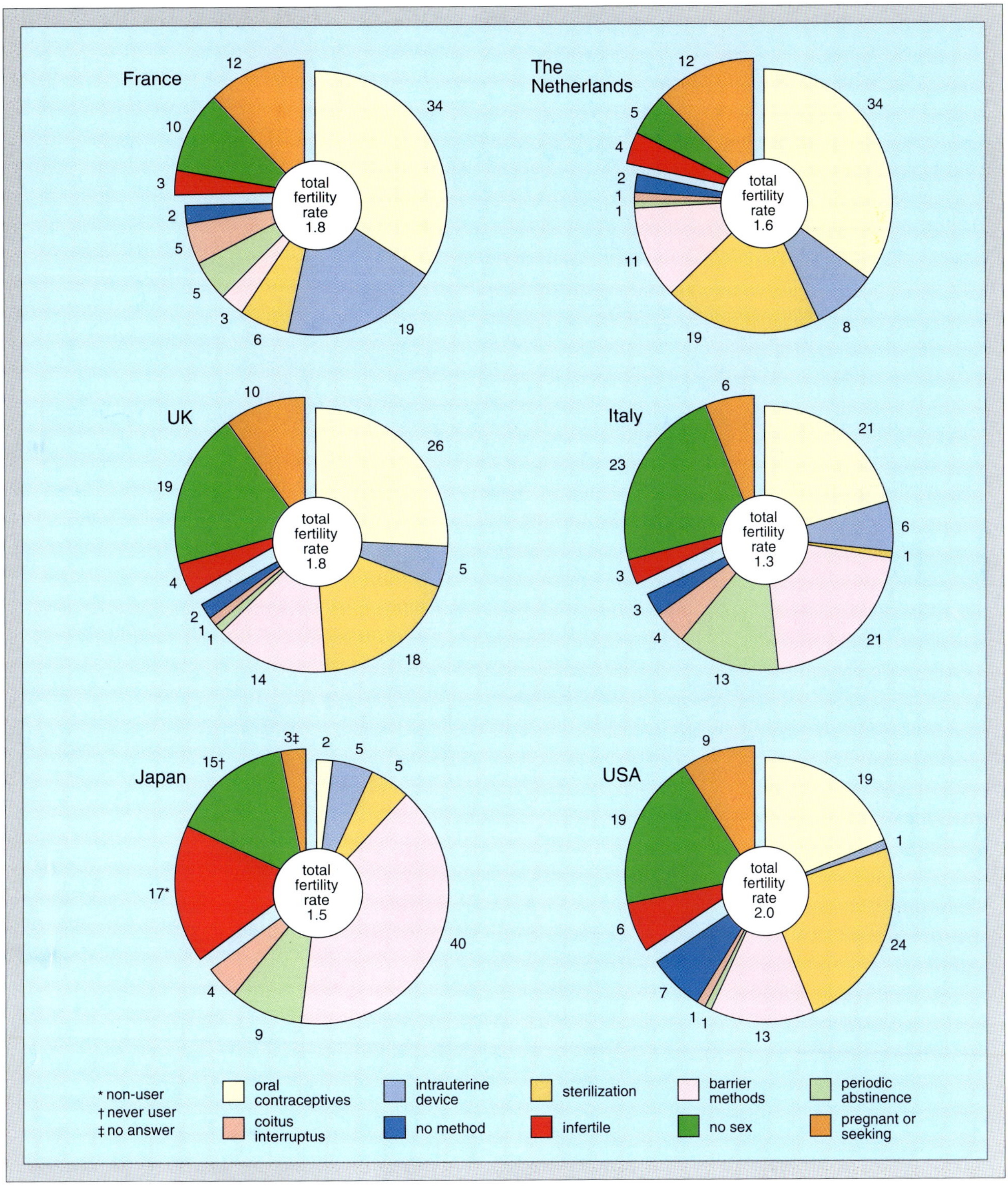

Figure 5.5 Current contraceptive use in women in selected countries (percentages)

Curative medicare	*Family planning*
Patient	User
Sickness	Health
Diagnosis by a health professional	Decision by user
Prescription of a therapy	Informed choice of method

Figure 5.6 Paradigms in disease and family planning

- Inappropriate eligibility criteria including age and parity
- Unwarranted contraindications
- Unnecessary process hurdles including lab tests
- Provider bias
- Restrictions on providers
- Regulatory barriers

Figure 5.7 Barriers to access to contraception

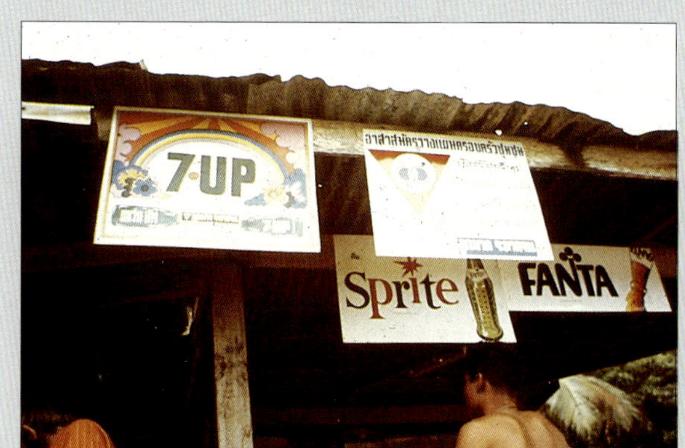

Figure 5.8 Condoms and pills are available in kiosks as part of the social marketing of the contraceptive program in Thailand

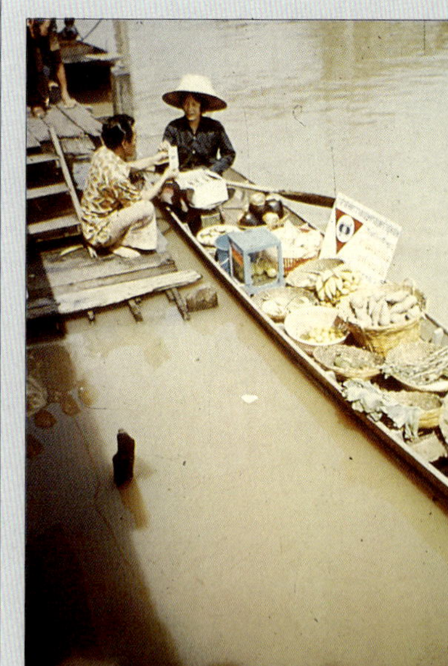

Figure 5.9 This lady travels the extensive Thai canalways stopping at homes by the canal to sell her wares, including contraceptives, providing 'door-to-door' sales

Rights of the client

Every family planning client has the right to:

1. Information
To learn about the benefits and availability of family planning

2. Access
To obtain services regardless of sex, creed, color, marital status or location

3. Choice
To decide freely whether to practice family planning and which method to choose

4. Safety
To be able to practice safe and effective family planning

5. Privacy
To have a private environment during counseling or services

6. Confidentiality
To be assured that any personal information will remain confidential

7. Dignity
To be treated with courtesy, consideration and attentiveness

8. Comfort
To feel comfortable when receiving services

9. Continuity
To receive contraceptive services and supplies for as long as needed

10. Opinion
To express views on the services offered

Figure 5.10 Rights of the client when seeking family planning advice. (Courtesy of the IPPF)

6

Hormonal contraception

'THE PILL'

The principle of oral contraceptives was clearly described in the 1920s by Ludwig Haberlandt in Austria, but oral contraceptives came to fruition only in the 1950s with the availability of cheap sources of orally effective ovarian hormones. Even then, it took the drive of Margaret Sanger and the generosity of Paige McCormack of International Harvesters to persuade scientists at the Worcester Foundation in Boston, Massachusetts, to conduct the necessary research; and the obstetrician John Rock, the reproductive physiologist Gregory Pincus and the scientist M. C. Chang to form a brilliant triumvirate which eventually provided women with a new and profoundly important contraceptive choice. In the way that IUDs were set back by the catastrophe of the Dalkon Shield, so oral contraceptives were unlucky in the timing and place of their origin. First, when the initial clinical trials were conducted in Massachusetts, contraceptives were still illegal under the old Comstock laws; for this reason, research was transferred to Puerto Rico. Second, in the late 1950s and early 1960s termination of pregnancy was unthinkable in the USA. In order to keep unintended pregnancies to a minimum, high doses of hormone were administered. An extraordinarily effective reversible contraceptive was produced with less than one pregnancy per 100 woman-years of exposure when correctly taken. However, follow-up soon showed that the high doses of hormone had some adverse effects.

The strengths and weaknesses of clinical trials and epidemiological studies of contraceptive effectiveness and safety are often misunderstood. Animal studies are difficult to interpret because of important differences in the reproductive systems of different species. Beagle dogs which have been used in long-term tests of steroids, for example, almost always develop breast cancer even when not exposed to artificial hormones. The type of clinical trials that are conducted prior to drug registration by the UK Committee on Safety of Medicines or the US Food and Drug Administration, or approval by the International Planned Parenthood Federation (IPPF) for use by member Family Planning Associations, usually provides a good measure of failure rates and insight into short-term side-effects – in the case of the pill, such things as nausea in the first few cycles of use and menstrual changes. Such trials, however, cannot detect rare events which might occur in one in 10 000, or even one in 1000 users. The introduction of new drugs and devices must be approached humbly and with caution but with an awareness that safety cannot be proved prior to widespread use.

Side-effects – good and bad

In the case of oral contraceptives, epidemiological studies in the UK in the second half of the 1960s showed that these drugs had an adverse effect on the cardiovascular system. Deep-vein thrombosis in the legs, heart attacks and strokes were all slightly more common in users of high-dose oral contraceptives. The risk to the woman, while genuine, was comparable to or lower than that associated with the pregnancies that would inevitably occur if a woman used a less effective method of contraception. In fact, risks associated with pill use are far lower than the risks taken almost daily when going about their normal activities (Figure 6.1). The only exception was among women who smoked; smoking and oral contraceptive use have a marked adverse interaction, particularly in women over the age of 35 years. Once these effects were understood, the dose of hormones was rapidly and successfully reduced and screening methods, particularly in relation to age and smoking, eliminated most of the risks. In large-scale studies conducted in the late 1980s of newer low-dose pills correctly used, there was little or no evidence of any adverse cardiovascular effect. Nevertheless, previous experience has left both women and physicians with a markedly pessimistic view of oral contraceptives. Studies from around the world show that the majority of women think that taking the pill is more dangerous than having a pregnancy (Figure 6.2) and very few are aware of the non-contraceptive benefits of using the pill (Figure 6.3).

The age of puberty, patterns of child-bearing and age of menopause all have a marked effect on the incidence of breast, uterine and ovarian cancer. Cervical cancer appears to be related primarily to the number of sexual partners, or to the number of sexual partners of the woman's husband. It was reasonable and necessary to explore the impact of oral contraceptives on reproductive cancers and many unfounded speculations were made in the early decades of use. In the later 1980s, several studies consistently showed that use of the pill had a marked protective effect against ovarian and endometrial cancer. The longer the pill is used, the greater the reduction in the chance of developing ovarian and uterine cancer. The protection lasts for 10–15 years after taking the last pill and may even last for a lifetime. As these two cancers also are less frequent in women who have multiple pregnancies and long intervals of lactation, it seems that the pill, by suppressing ovulation, brings about the same pattern of protection.

The commonest reproductive cancer is that of the breast, which in the USA strikes one in 11 women and kills one in 18. Cancer of the breast has become more common in every decade in the twentieth century and the vast majority of women who have suffered this scourge of death and illness have been too old ever to have taken oral contraceptives. When all the women who have used the pill are compared with non-users, then no adverse or beneficial effect of the pill in relation to breast cancer has been demonstrated (Figure 6.4). In the small group of women who are unfortunate enough to develop breast cancer before the age of 35 years, and who also used the pill early in their reproductive life, some studies show a slight increase in risk while others show no effect. It is also possible that the first pregnancy is associated with a *slight* short-term rise in the risk of breast cancer, followed by a longer-term statistically more significant protective effect.

After 30 years of use and with 75 million current users and an equal or greater number of women who have used the pill in the past, a vast and sometimes overwhelming amount of information exists: the pill may be the best-studied medication in the twentieth century. When all the material from various sources is put together, then it seems that in younger women (whether they smoke or not), the protection against ovarian/uterine cancer more than outweighs any cardiovascular risk attributable to low-dose pills. If an adverse effect on breast cancer risk in younger women is ever confirmed, this will reduce but not totally eliminate the overall protection against malignancy. In older women, particularly those who smoke, cardiovascular disease risk may slightly outweigh the cancer protection. At all levels of analysis, the risks are very small.

One way of expressing a combination of risks and benefits is to use a computer model to calculate the impact on overall expectation of life. For a woman who takes the pill early in her reproductive years, the drug may prolong her life by 3 or 4 days, on average, while one who takes the pill later in life may shorten her life by 10 or 20 days; for comparison, an individual who smokes a pack of cigarettes a day reduces their average expectation of life by over 4 years. Another way of looking at pill risk is to point out that even the old high-dose pills carried less risk than smoking *one* cigarette a day. The recommendation that the pill should be in slot machines and cigarettes on prescription remains a sound one.

Recently, there have been suggestions in both the USA and UK that oral contraceptives should be switched from their current prescription status to over-the-counter items, like the condom.

WORLDWIDE USE

The main forms of oral contraception currently available include the combined oral contraceptives containing both estrogen and progestogen, the progestogen-only pill and the hormonal postcoital pill; the latter at the present time is reserved for emergency use only.

Pill use in different countries of the world varies a great deal and estimates may not reveal the true picture. Rates of usage can vary from 2% in Japan to 34% in The Netherlands. The factors which determine pill use include biological factors such as family size and age; effect of the media; religion; medical, legal and political aspects of the family planning program in the country; and the availability and number of outlets where the pill can be obtained.

The most widely used oral preparations are those containing estrogen and progestogen taken in constant amount for 20, 21 or 22 days followed by an interval without steroids during which uterine bleeding occurs. The commonest regimen is a 21-day course, followed by an interval of 7 days when no tablet is taken, or placebo, iron and/or vitamin tablets are substituted. The tendency in recent years has been to reduce the dose of both estrogen and progestogen, with some currently available preparations having the minimum effective dose.

Phasic preparations, with a changing dose of progestogen, allow the use of smaller amounts of steroids while still maintaining good cycle control. These pills try to mimic the normal cycle and have an initial estrogen dominance. They require slightly more compliance in use.

COMBINED ORAL CONTRACEPTIVES

Today's low-dose combined oral contraceptives contain less than 50 μg estrogen, down from 150 μg in the first oral contraceptive and 50–100 μg in those of the late 1960s and the 1970s. Estrogen doses of 20–35 μg ethinylestradiol are the most common. Some low-dose pills use 50 μg mestranol, which is roughly as potent as 35 μg ethinylestradiol. Progestin doses also have dropped substantially. For example, doses of norethindrone have dropped from 10 mg to 1.0 or 0.5 mg. Because progestins vary in potency by weight, doses of other progestins range from 0.05 to 2.0 mg.

Low-estrogen oral contraceptives are now the most widely used. Data from 37 countries in 1987 suggest that low-estrogen pills accounted for nearly 85% of pharmacy sales of oral contraceptives in the developed countries and almost 60% in the developing countries. In 1988 they comprised almost 80% of oral contraceptives donated to family planning programs in developing countries.

Mode of action

The primary action of combined oral contraceptive pills is the cessation of ovulation brought about by the inhibition of pituitary follicle stimulating hormone, thus inhibiting follicular maturation in the ovary, and by the abolition of the estrogen-mediated positive feedback, which is the physiological trigger for the ovulatory surge of luteinizing hormone (Figures 6.5 and 6.6). Cervical mucus is affected mainly by progestogen and rendered inhospitable to sperm. The receptivity of the endometrium to the blastocyst is also reduced. These latter two mechanisms act as a back-up to the main ovarian effect.

ADVANTAGES AND DISADVANTAGES

When choosing a method of contraception a potential user must have access to up-to-date objective information on advantages and disadvantages. The pill has a number of short-term advantages and disadvantages which users should understand (Figures 6.7 and 6.8, respectively). The longer-term non-contraceptive benefits of the combined oral contraceptive pill are outlined in Figure 6.3. Women using the pill have a flattened endometrium and, therefore, the periods are both regular and less in volume than in women who do not use hormonal contraceptives.

Over the years and partly propelled by medicolegal considerations, the US Food and Drug Administration and other drug national regulatory authorities have required manufacturers to provide useful information about benefits of oral contraceptive use. Side-effects and contraindications to pill use are outlined in Figures 6.8 and 6.9.

The pill is only effective if taken correctly and consistently. Many studies have shown, however, that many users are not fully aware of what they should do if they forget to take a pill or delay taking it, and also what should be done if the user has diarrhea or vomits the pill (Figure 6.10).

If users forget to take the pill, then loss of efficacy may be pronounced for the next 7 days or more if pills are omitted early in a packet. The 14-day rule shown below is supported by the evidence available and is easy to convey to pill takers.

The 14-day rule

(1) If pill taking has been delayed by less than 12 h, then the missed pill should be taken, the next one should be taken on time, and no loss of contraception should be assumed.

(2) If there is a delay of more than 12 h in taking any pill, especially the first in the packet, then the missed pill should be taken, or if more than one, then the last two missed pills.

   (a) The regular pill-taking routine should be resumed.

   (b) Extra precautions should be taken (e.g. the sheath) for the next 14 days, through the pill-free week, and into the start of the next packet if necessary.

PROGESTOGEN-ONLY PILLS

The progestogen-only pills are estrogen-free oral contraceptives containing a microdose of progestogen either from the norethindrone or levonorgestrel group. The first progestogen-only pill was introduced in 1969.The progestogen-only pill has to be taken daily and at a regular time without a 7-day break. It may make it easier for women to adhere to a regular pill-taking pattern.

The efficacy of the progestogen-only pill is less than that of the combined oral contraceptive. Failure rates vary between 0.3 and 5.0 per 100 woman-years. They exert their main action on the cervical mucus, leading to the production of thick mucus with poor sperm penetrability.

The main side-effect of the progestogen-only pill is an irregular bleeding cycle, and in some women amenorrhea can result.

Progestogen-only pills combine good efficiency with lack of major side-effects and minimal alteration in metabolic effects. They may be particularly suitable for women who have side-effects or contraindications to the combined oral contraceptives, in particular those side-effects believed to be estrogen-related. Progestogen-only pills are suitable for older women, mainly over the age of 40 years, who are non-smokers, and for women during lactation.

Emergency (postcoital) use of the pill

Many postcoital techniques to prevent pregnancy after unprotected intercourse can be found in ancient writings. For instance, in France in the eighteenth century, a postcoital douche was available in every good hotel, and in Persia in the eighth century postcoital sneezing and jumping backward the magical seven steps were supposed to dislodge the semen. Nowadays, the uselessness of such methods is recognized.

Emergency (postcoital) contraception using orally administered hormones has been shown to be considered as a one-time procedure and not a routine approach to contraception. The commonly used preparations are oral contraceptives containing 50 μg ethinylestradiol and 0.25 mg levonorgestrel (other similar formulations also have high efficacy). Two tablets should be taken within 24 h of intercourse, followed by two more tablets 12 h later.

This method is suitable for women exposed to unprotected sexual intercourse. It is effective only if instituted within 72 h of exposure. Standard contraindications to the use of combined hormonal contraceptives should be observed. Possible side-effects include nausea, vomiting, irregular uterine bleeding, breast tenderness and headache.

The woman should be seen a month later for counseling for elective contraception and to exclude the possibility of pregnancy.

LONG-ACTING HORMONAL METHODS

Injectables

Ovarian hormones are more easily delivered systemically than orally. A comparison of the effects of the combined pill, the progestogen-only pill and injectable preparations is shown in Figure 6.11, and the mechanism of action of injectables is shown in Figure 6.12. The problem with injectables is how to obtain a regular release over a long interval of time. The two most commonly used intramuscular injectable preparations are a 3-monthly injection of a relatively high dose of medroxyprogesterone acetate (150 mg in a microcrystalline suspension; DMPA, Depo-Provera®, Megestron®) and a 2-monthly injection of norethindrone enanthate (200 mg in oil; NET-OEN®, Noristerat®, Norigest®). Depo-Provera has an exceptionally low failure rate (under 1%) but it also takes some time to eliminate all the hormone after the last injection and there is some delay in the return of fertility, although there is no evidence of any long-term impairment. Norethindrone enanthate uses a slightly lower dose of progestogen but is less tolerant of delays between injections, and the injection needs to be repeated after 2 rather than 3 months. Contraindications of long-acting preparations include hypertension, diabetes and large fibroids; side-effects include irregular bleeding, amenorrhea, delayed return of ovulation, hypertension and changes in carbohydrate metabolism. As these preparations lack estrogens, they appear to have no adverse effect on the cardiovascular system. They should not be used if there is a suspicion of pregnancy.

Until recently, monthly injectable formulations were only available in China and some Latin American countries. They usually contain lower doses of a long-acting progestogen and a small dose of a shorter-acting estrogen, which gives rise to regular bleeding. Examples of this type of formulation include:

(1) Norethindrone enanthate 50 mg + estradiol valerate 5 mg;

(2) Depot medroxyprogesterone acetate 25 mg + estradiol cypionate 4 mg;

(3) Dihydroxyprogesterone acetophenide 150 mg + estradiol enanthate 10 mg.

The World Health Organization has recently developed a monthly injectable – Cyclofem® – combining an already known progestogen, depot medroxyprogesterone acetate 25 mg and a known estrogen, estradiol cypionate 5 mg. This has been available in Mexico, Thailand and in Indonesia from 1993 and is likely to be used in many other countries. In addition, a once-a-month injectable Mesigyna® containing norethindrone enanthate 50mg and estradiol valerate 5mg is also now available. These are highly effective contraceptives which achieve a better cycle control than the longer-acting injectables. However, monthly injectables have the disadvantage of requiring more frequent administration. In order to prevent spread of infection when giving injectable contraceptives, health-workers are advised to use disposable syringes and needles. However, due to costs and shortage of syringes and needles many developing countries continue to reuse equipment, and thus the spread of infection is known to take place. To eliminate the problem of reusing needles and syringes, a single-use prefilled syringe for long-term injectables has been developed (Figure 6.13).

Injectable use has been literally dogged by adverse headlines coming from studies on Depo-Provera given to beagle dogs, and as a result many women who would have benefited greatly from its use have been denied the choice. When the drug industry first started doing long-term cancer studies in animals in the 1950s and 1960s they chose beagle dogs for no better reason than the fact that they are good-natured and tolerate laboratory routines without biting the attendants! Physiologically they were a disastrous choice. They happen to be a species in which, even without any intervention, there is a high rate of spontaneous breast cancer. Unlike human beings, where reproduction is independent of the season, bitches are seasonal breeding animals and the sexual cycle is fairly different from that of primates. The occurrence of breast cancer in beagles given high doses of Depo-Provera confused scientists and alarmed the public. Sincere consumer groups argued that the method was dangerous and in particular should not be given to women in poor countries.

Beagle dogs are no longer required as test animals by any national drug regulatory authority. Injectable contraceptives have been licenced in the majority of the world's countries, from Chile to Britain to Thailand to New Zealand. Large-scale case–control studies of women with cancer in Third World countries have shown injectables behave like oral contraceptives. Like the pill, injectable contraceptives probably reduce the risk of ovarian and uterine cancer and, as they lack the estrogenic effects, they may, overall, be even safer. In 1992, the expert committee advising the US Food and Drug Administration once again recommended approval of Depo-Provera as a contraceptive for USA women, and finally, 28 years after the first recommendation (1965), Depo-Provera became available to USA women as a contraceptive. Undoubtedly, a great many women have died from childbirth and abortion whose lives might have been saved had injectable contraceptives been fully understood at an early stage in their history.

Long-acting injectable contraceptives are highly effective. Serum iron levels are noted to be increased during use of these drugs. The advantages are listed in Figure 6.14. The disadvantages, on the other hand, are relatively few. They cause a change in menstrual patterns, inducing amenorrhea or spotting. A potential disadvantage is the inability to withdraw the drug promptly. There is also the potential for abuse by health practitioners who do not always tell the user all the disadvantages. Once the injection has been given, the woman has no control over the method, other than to wait until the effects wear off. Long-acting injectables are not practical for self-administration.

Injectable biodegradable polymer systems are being developed in which particles – microspheres, microcapsules or polymeric powder – are injected; these involve an inert drug carrier and allow a controlled rate of drug release.

Implants

Subcutaneous implants with constant slow release of a variety of different progestogens have been shown to provide excellent contraception. These have usually consisted of silastic capsules packed with crystalline steroid. Attempts are also being made to perfect a biodegradable polymer which will allow constant steroid release as the polymer is absorbed. The 5-year levonorgestrel-releasing system (NORPLANT®) developed by the Population Council is now available in many countries (Figures 6.15–6.18).

Under local anesthetic and using a small incision, the implant is inserted under the skin. It is effective within 24 h of insertion and has a 5-year duration of action with constant release. There are no estrogen-related effects. Removal is possible, and the implant is safe, effective and well-liked.

The woman should, however, be fully counseled. She should be told what side-effects to expect and also be told that she can, and has a right to, have the implant removed at any time, if she is unhappy about the method due to side-effects or if she wants the implant removed for other reasons. Side-effects are similar to those found with long-acting progestogen-only contraceptives and include irregular bleeding, amenorrhea and occasional weight change.

The removal procedure takes a little longer than the insertion procedure. Also, the health care providers have to be trained properly in both procedures of insertion and removal. The health care provider should be trained in counseling and should know that a woman has a right to request removal and that her wishes should be complied with.

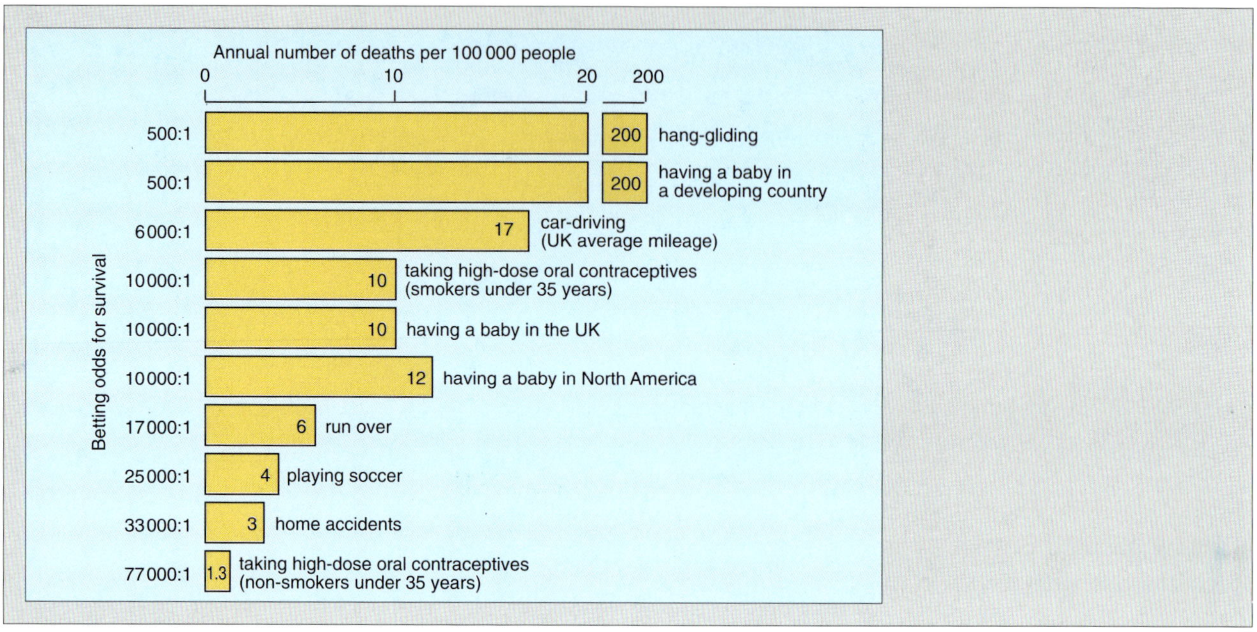

Figure 6.1 Pill risks compared with other risks women run. These risks are lower, and possibly eliminated in the low-dose oral contraceptives now in widespread use. (Adapted from Guillebaud, J. (1987). *The Pill*, 3rd edn. (Oxford: Oxford University Press))

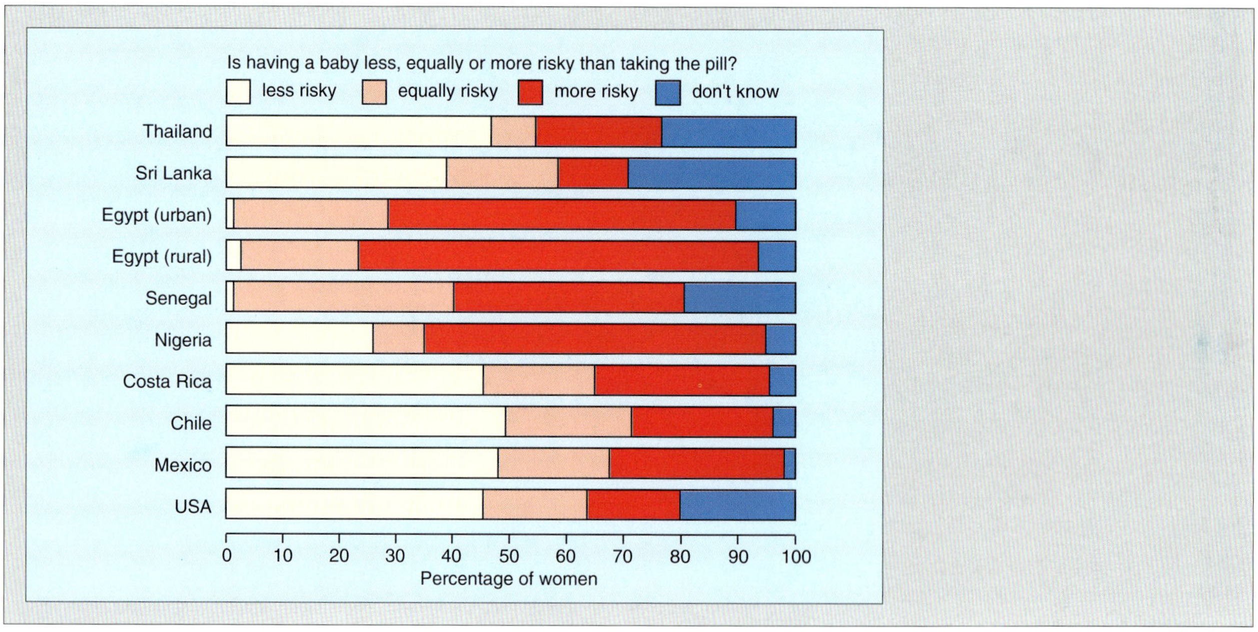

Figure 6.2 The majority of women think taking the pill is more dangerous than having a pregnancy. (Source, Family Health International (1987))

The incidence of the following conditions is reduced:

- Ovarian cancer
- Endometrial cancer
- Pelvic inflammatory disease
- Ectopic pregnancy
- Iron deficiency anemia
- Primary dysmenorrhea
- Benign breast disease
- Functional ovarian cysts

Potential benefits include protection against:

- Osteoporosis
- Toxic shock syndrome
- Leiomyomata
- Rheumatoid arthritis

Figure 6.3 Non-contraceptive benefits of the combined oral contraceptive pill

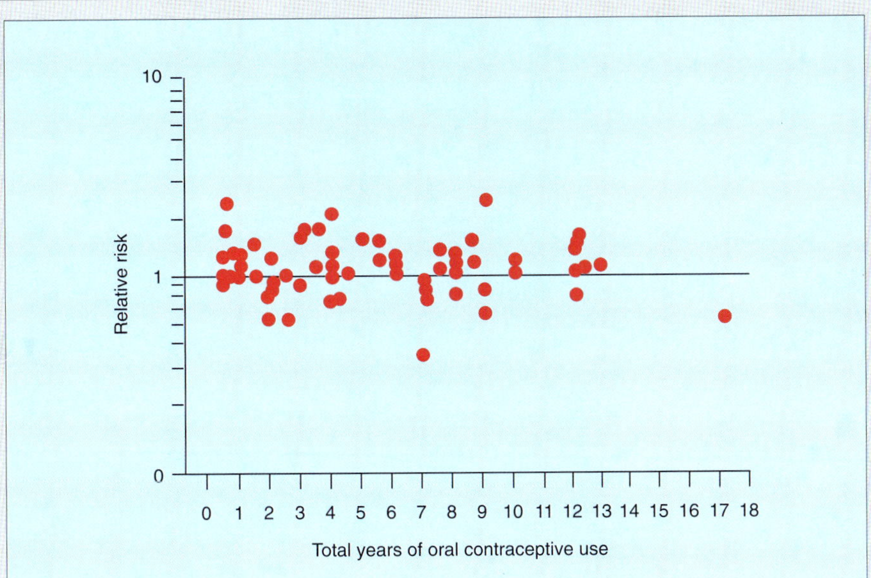

Figure 6.4 Breast cancer in women younger than 60 years of age: relative risk by total years of oral contraceptive use in 17 studies since 1980

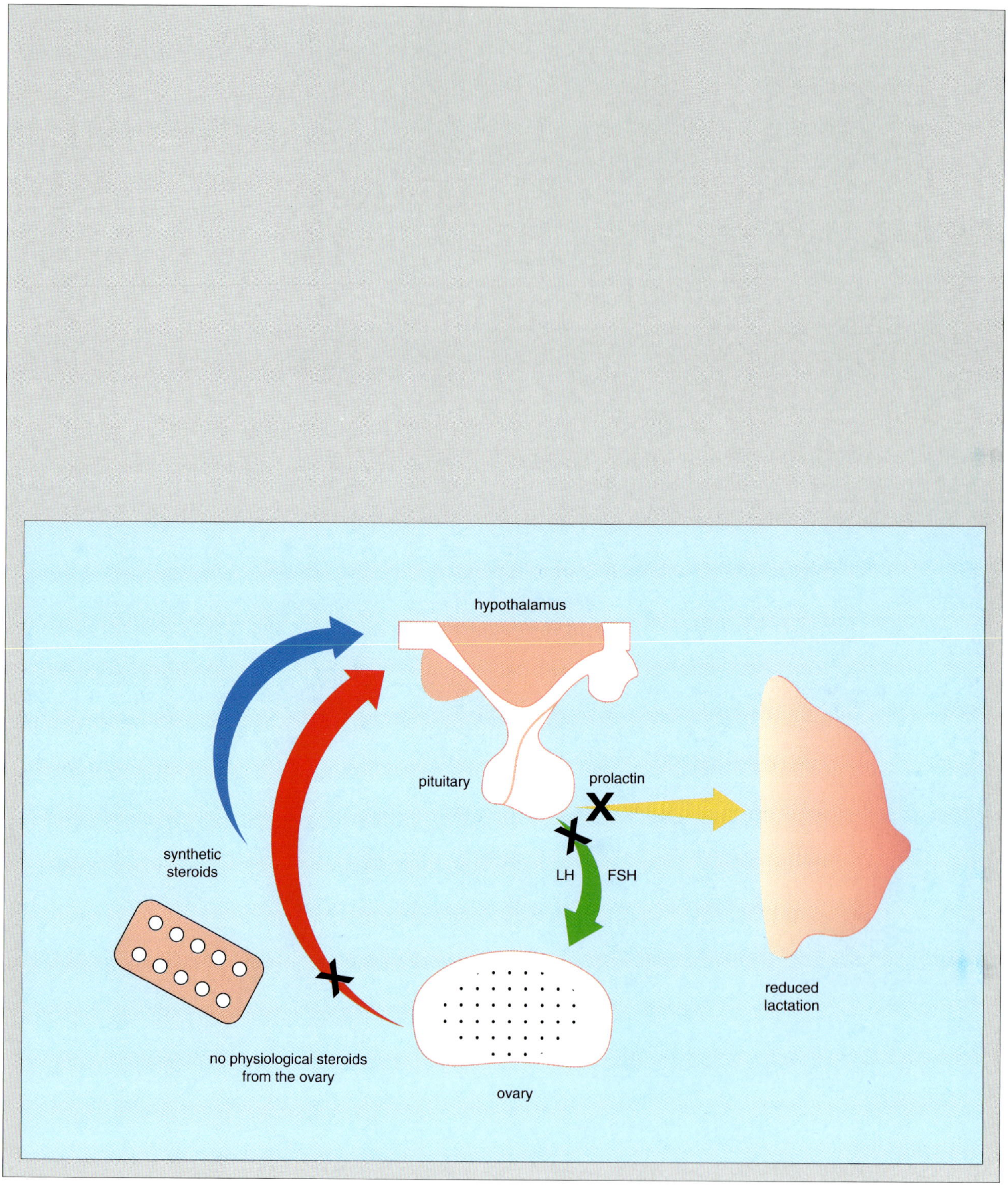

Figure 6.5 Alteration of hormonal cycles by oral contraception

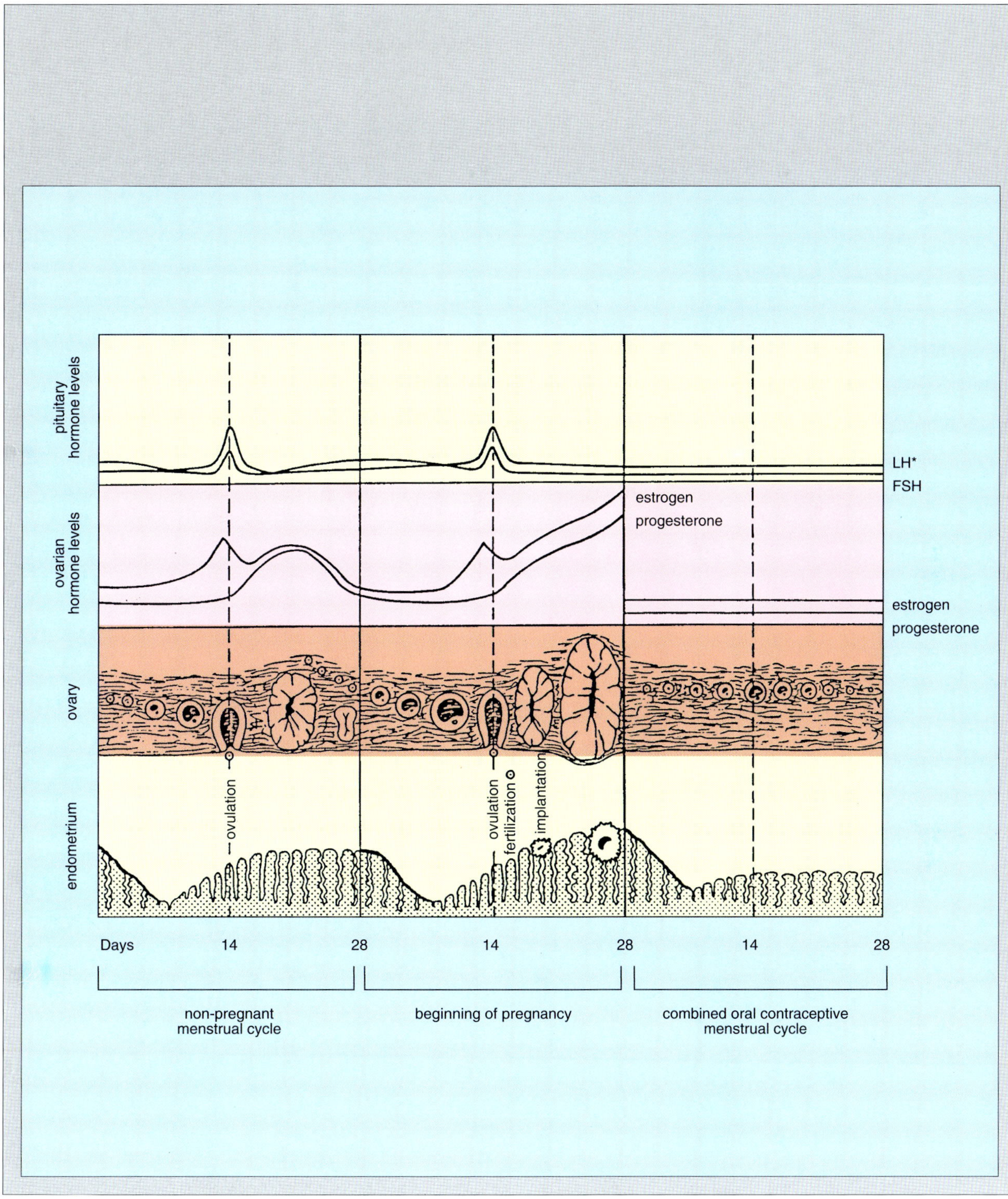

Figure 6.6 A diagrammatic comparison showing changes which occur in the endometrium, ovary and in plasma hormone levels during the non-pregnant menstrual cycle, the beginning of pregnancy, and the oral contraceptive menstrual cycle. LH, luteinizing hormone; FSH, follicle stimulating hormone. (Adapted from *Expecting a Baby*. (London: BBC Publications))

- Acne is improved with some pills
- Breast tenderness is usually reduced
- 100% protection against pregnancy is assured
- Intercourse is unaffected
- Regular menstruation
- Timing of menstruation can be controled
- No ovulation pain
- Less premenstrual tension
- Less period pain
- Less heavy bleeding, therefore less anemia
- Less pelvic infection
- 100% reversible

Figure 6.7 Short-term advantages of the combined oral contraceptive pill

- Amenorrhea
- Mid-cycle spotting
- Depression
- Fluid retention/bloatedness
- Headaches
- Reduced libido in some users
- Migraine
- Nausea in the first month of use
- Weight gain

Figure 6.8 Short-term disadvantages of the combined oral contraceptive pill

Absolute contraindications	*Temporary absolute contraindications*
• Past or present thrombophlebitis or thromboembolic disorders • Cerebrovascular or coronary artery disease • Malignancy of the breast • Malignancy of the cervix, uterus or ovaries • Focal migraine	• Known or suspected pregnancy until non-pregnant • Undiagnosed abnormal genital tract bleeding until diagnosis is clear, particularly to exclide malignancy • Acute liver disease such as infectious hepatitis until liver function tests are normal

Figure 6.9 Contraindications of combined oral contraception

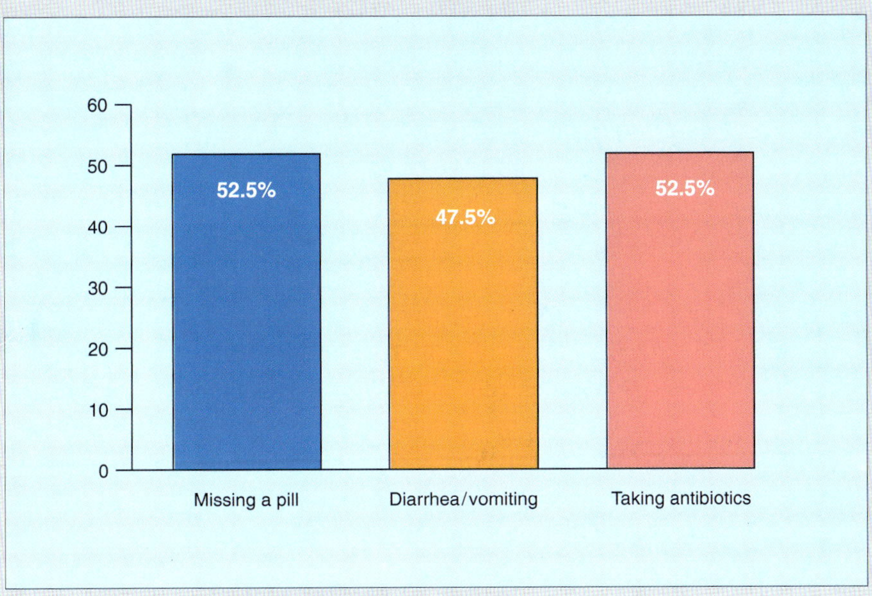

Figure 6.10 Percentage of users of the pill who are unaware of the consequences of missing a pill, if antibiotics are being taken, or if diarrhea and/or vomiting is occurring. (Source, Family Health International)

Effects	*Combined pill*	*Progestogen-only pill*	*Injectable*
Ovulation suppressed	yes	no	yes
Endometrial changes	yes	yes	yes
Cervical mucus changes	yes	yes	yes
Lactation suppressed	yes	no	no
Pregnancy rate per woman-years in use	0.5–5.0	2–10	1.0

Figure 6.11 Comparison of action of contraceptive hormone preparations

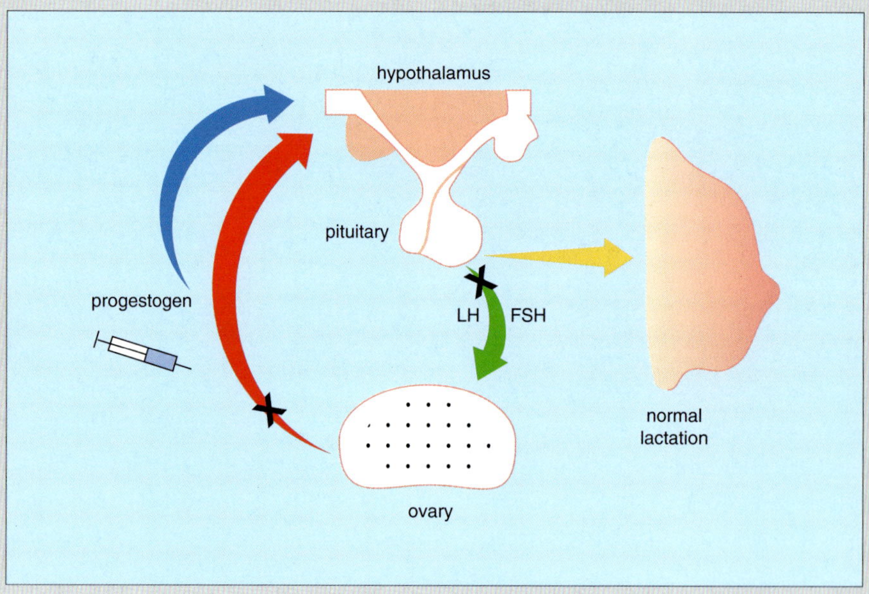

Figure 6.12 Alteration of hormonal cycles by injectables

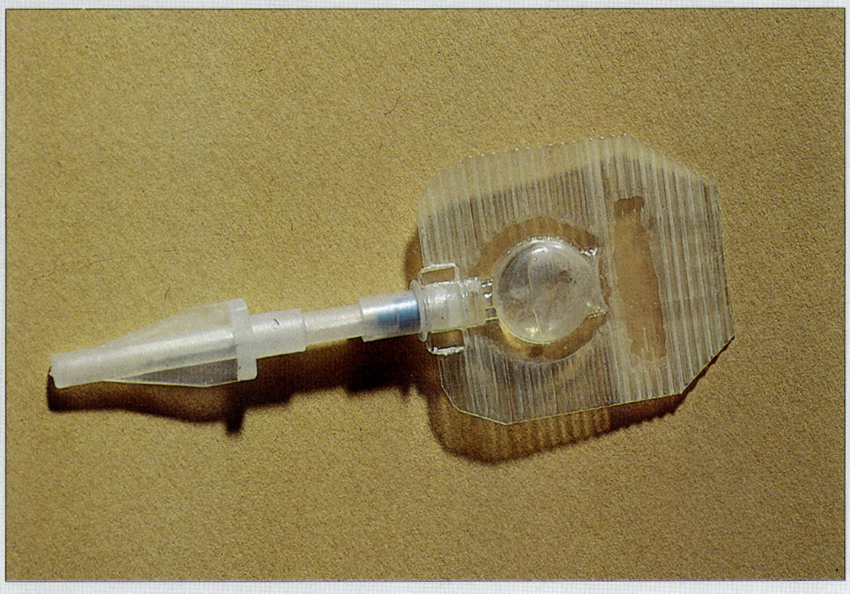

Figure 6.13 An example of a single-use prefilled syringe. It can be used for long-acting injectable contraceptives. (Courtesy of The Program for Applied Technology in Health)

- Postinjection infertility lasting 4–9 months
- No known interference with lactation
- No increased risk of cancer
- Protection against pelvic inflammatory disease
- Protection against ovarian/endometrial cancer
- No estrogen-related side-effects
- Elimination of user error (i.e. user compliance not a factor)
- Use is not coitus-related
- Infrequent administration – an advantage in prolonged use
- High degree of privacy (no supplies need to be kept around the house)
- A clinical setting is not required for provision of this method of contraception
- Injectables are acceptable forms of medication in many cultures
- Absorption of the drug is not dependent on normal gastrointestinal function
- Pregnancy rates are low
- No mortality has been associated with their use

Figure 6.14 Advantages of long-acting contraceptives

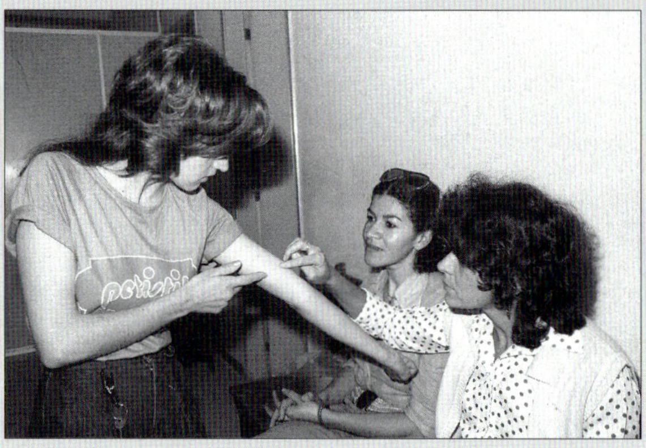

Figure 6.15 Volunteer in Brazil showing position for implantation of NORPLANT capsules. (Source, Population Council, New York, USA)

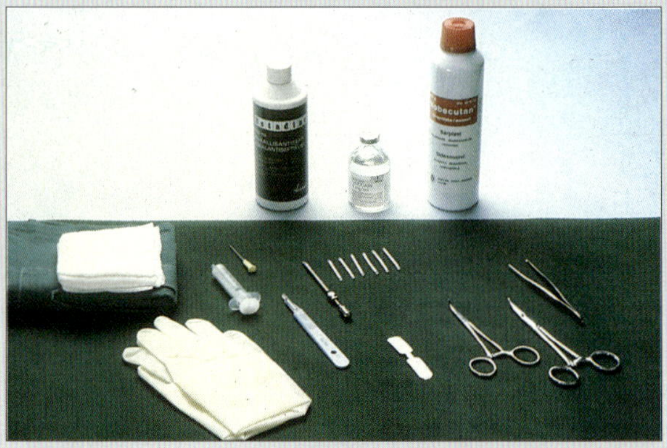

Figure 6.16 The simple equipment necessary for implantation of the NORPLANT capsules. (Source, Population Council, New York, USA)

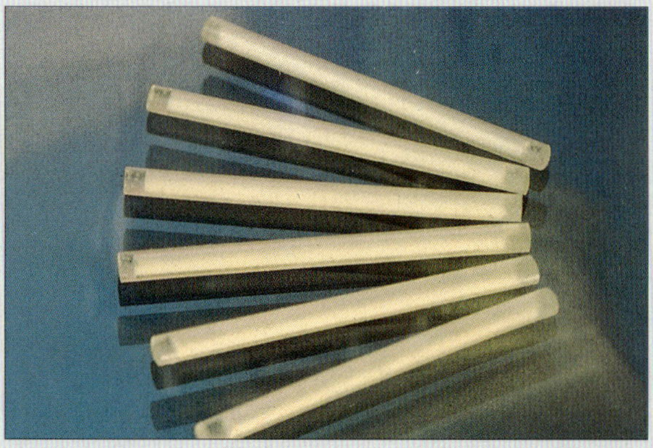

Figure 6.17 The silastic capsules of the NORPLANT implant. (Source, Population Council, New York, USA)

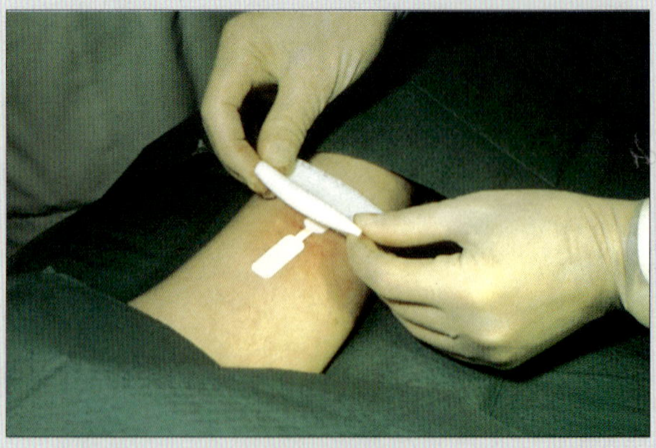

Figure 6.18 The arm after implantation of NORPLANT. (Source, Population Council, New York, USA)

7

Condoms

Condoms are a common-sense method of contraception with a long history. The fifteenth century anatomist Gabriel Fallopius, who first described the uterine tubes which still carry his name, described the use of chemically impregnated silk sheaths. His work involved one of the first clinical trials in the history of medicine and, interestingly, he described use of the device after coitus. The word condom is sometimes ascribed to Dr Condom of the Court of Charles II, who was so worried about the number of illegitimate children fathered by the King that he invented the device. This story is probably apocryphal; a more likely derivation of the name is from the Latin 'condus' for 'receptacle'.

Condoms became a widespread family planning method only in the twentieth century. Prior to that, they were used principally for the prevention of sexually transmissible infections. An advertisement for condoms in 1796 read:

> To guard yourself from shame or fear,
> Votaries to Venus hasten here,
> None in my ware e'er found a flaw,
> Self-preservation's Nature's law.

Britain appears to have been the first country to commercialize the sale of condoms. Initially, sheaths were made from animal membranes and in the USA 'natural skins' are still sold as luxury items. They are made from the ceca of Australian sheep, removed in the slaughterhouse and cleaned and then shipped to the Caribbean where small elastic rings are sewn into the open ends before they are packaged and sold in the USA.

Rubber condoms became possible after the vulcanization of rubber was first carried out by Hancock and Goodyear in 1844. In the second half of the nineteenth century hand-dipped devices were made and in the twentieth century large-scale mass production (Figure 7.1) and quality control of high quality rubber condoms (Figure 7.2) were devised. Major manufacturers are in Japan, Western Europe and the USA. A relatively small number of manufacturers control production and most of the sales also go through relatively few distributors. Although there are no specific monopolistic practices, new manufacturers find it difficult to break into the market and profit margins are relatively high.

As noted earlier, there are biological reasons why we are all innately shy about human sexual intercourse and therefore coy about contraception (see p. 40). Condoms have long been perceived as a shameful and an under-the-counter product. One way of defusing embarrassment is through humor; therefore, anthropomorphic penises putting on condoms have become an increasingly widespread educational device, appearing on T-shirts from Sweden to Thailand. Simple illustrations of the correct use of condoms are provided by many organizations around the world. Family Health International owns a 77 000 cubic foot non-lubricated nipple-ended hot-air balloon. For some people it is the ultimate symbol of all that is embarrassing about family planning. It is notable that the Guinness Book of Records has never acknowledged an application for its inclusion. Its use was banned in North Carolina but was accepted in Montreal – providing any written message that it carried was translated into French!

Condoms were the major artificial method of family planning in the UK until the second half of the twentieth century and they remain the commonest method in Japan. Condoms have no significant side-effects. The most common reason for failure is probably non-use, although it is also important to remember that latex is very easily damaged by petroleum-based or other greasy lubricants. Condoms illustrate the difficulty of assessing contraceptive failure rates. The normal measure is the number of pregnancies per 100 woman-years of exposure (e.g. 100 women using the method for 1 year or 20 women for 5 years). There have been relatively few studies of condom use and those that do exist have not been conducted to the exacting standards of modern clinical trials. When couples have used condoms for many years, they often achieve failure rates of well under five pregnancies per 100 woman-years of exposure. But those who are not familiar with the method make many more mistakes.

When assessing the failure rate of any method of contraception, it is rarely useful to quote an exact number but more informative to give a range of failure rates. It is easy to establish a rank order for effectiveness of methods of contraception (Figure 7.3), with condoms being more effective than coitus interruptus and oral contraceptives more effective than condoms. However, there still will be people who probably would use the pill less well than the condom, or vice versa.

For several decades, those working in family planning have tried to separate the use of condoms for contraception from their use for protection against sexually transmitted diseases. With the spread of AIDS, condoms are once again becoming a significant, life-saving item. Latex condoms have a limited shelf-life. They are greatly weakened (within 30 seconds) by contact with oil-based as opposed to aqueous lubricants. Even when purchased in bulk, a year's supply is more expensive than oral contraceptives.

No one disputes that sexually transmitted infections represent a major public health problem in the world today. The probability of sexually transmitted diseases increases with increasing number of sexual partners. It should be pointed out that the use of a barrier contraceptive will reduce the risk of certain diseases. However, the condom can give a false sense of security since it does not prevent the spread of all infections.

Good quality latex condoms are impervious to bacteria. Testing using a bacteriophage, similar in size to HIV and combined with simulated coitus, found significant leakage with some brands. Condoms made from animal membranes are permeable to viruses.

Clinical studies show that latex condoms offer substantial protection against herpes simplex, *Chlamydia trachomatis*, cytomegalovirus, *Neisseria gonorrhoeae* and *Ureaplasma urealyticum*.

In a study of USA seamen in the Philippines, no man who reported using condoms while in post became infected with gonorrhea.

People should use more condoms for two reasons – to prevent unwanted pregnancy and to save lives. Yet, in 1990, condoms were used only half as often as needed – in total, approximately 6 000 million worldwide. However, by a rough estimate, condoms were actually needed in more than 13 000 million acts of sexual intercourse that risked unwanted pregnancy, AIDS and/or other sexually transmissible disease. Figure 7.4 shows the use of condoms among married women of reproductive age in various countries.

The public health challenge today is therefore to try to ensure that condoms are used each and every time they are needed. This task is not simple, easy or quick. But it is urgent and important. Action is needed in four broad areas as indicated in Figure 7.5, and in order to increase condom use, policy-makers should take the steps illustrated in Figure 7.6.

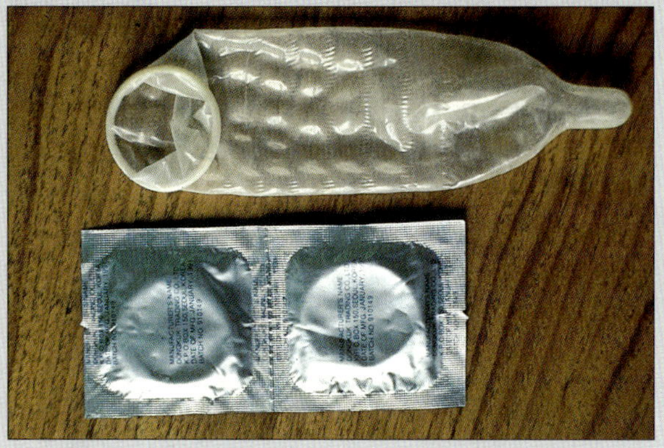

Figure 7.1 An example of a high quality rubber condom

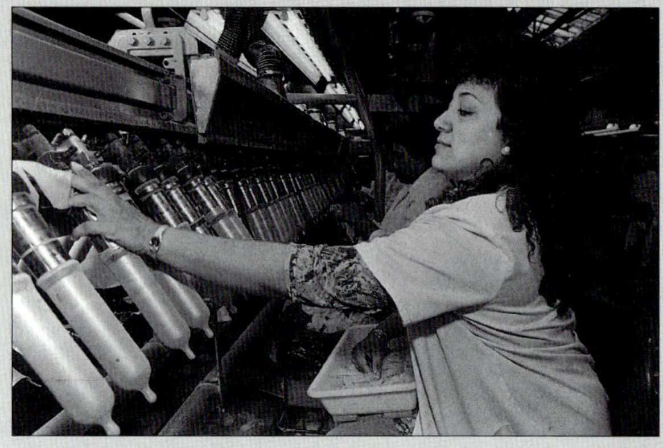

Figure 7.2 Electronic testing of condoms (Durex – London Rubber Company factory (London International))

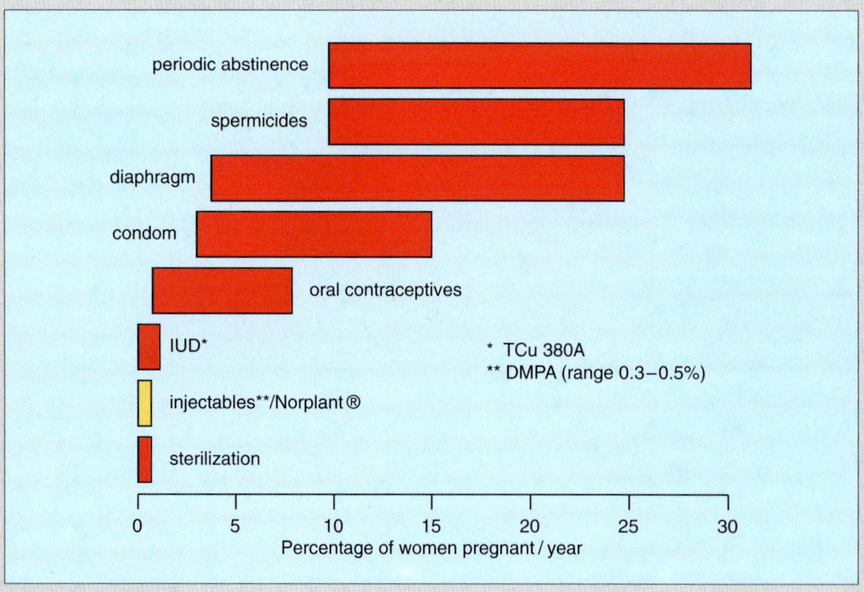

Figure 7.3 Range of failure rates for different methods of contraception

Region and Country	Number	Year	% using any method	% of contraceptors using condoms
Asia and Pacific				
Bangladesh	238	1985	25	7
China	58 426	1988	77	3
Indonesia	166	1987	48	3
Korea (Rep. of)	383	1985	70	10
Pakistan	383	1984–85	8	22
Thailand	56	1987	68	2
Latin America & Caribbean				
Brazil	16	1986	66	3
Costa Rica	75	1986	70	19
El Salvador	92	1988	47	5
Paraguay	383	1987	45	5
Near East & North Africa				
Egypt	91	1988	38	6
Turkey	144	1988	63	11
Developed countries				
France	206	1988	72	6
Japan	383	1986	64	69
United States	248	1988	74	14
West Germany	87	1985	78	7

Figure 7.4 Use of condoms among married couples of reproductive age in various countries

- Promoting condoms to the public
- Informing and counseling people so that they may use condoms consistently and correctly
- Making condoms universally available at affordable prices
- Manufacturing more condoms as demand grows

Figure 7.5 The four broad areas in which action needs to be taken to ensure that condoms are used every time they are needed

- Eliminate all barriers to import or manufacture, including duties and taxes
- Make increasing condom use a top public health priority
- Encourage innovative distribution, such as employment-based programs, social marketing programs, community-based distribution and school-based programs
- Eliminate policy and legal barriers to condom promotion

Figure 7.6 Initiatives which should be taken by the policy makers to increase the use of condoms

8

Female barrier contraception and spermicides

BARRIER CONTRACEPTION

In the early nineteenth century, experiments began with a variety of cervical and vaginal barriers, several of which are in current use. The greatest appeal of barrier methods is also their greatest drawback: they have no apparent effects on the human system and need to be used only at the time of intercourse. However, they are less effective than other methods. They should be used with a spermicide, as this improves effectiveness.

A number of chemicals kill sperm. The most commonly used is a detergent called nonoxynol-9. Spermicides can be used alone or in combination with a barrier such as a diaphragm. Spermicides can be formulated as pessaries, gels, foams from an aerosol can, or in the form of a water-soluble film (Figure 8.1). Most spermicides also kill a number of pathogens and clinical studies show that the regular use of spermicides reduces the risk of gonorrhea and *Chlamydia* infection. In high doses, or in sensitive individuals spermicides can damage the vaginal epithelium or even cause penile irritation. Recent studies suggest at certain doses nonoxynol-9 may prove a useful protection against HIV/AIDS.

Sponges of various shapes and types have been available for many years. Disposable plastic sponges, such as the Today® sponge, impregnated with a spermicide, were first marketed in the 1980s (Figure 8.2).

The cervical cap was invented in the early nineteenth century and caps were on sale in New York in the 1860s, but they were not approved by the US Food and Drugs Administration until the 1980s. It is a small thimble-shaped device of rubber or metal that fits directly around the cervix. It should form an airtight seal and is held in place by suction. A small quantity of spermicide is applied before insertion, and the cap can be left in position for several days.

The diaphragm (Figures 8.3 and 8.4) is a dome-shaped rubber device which is inserted into the vagina and covers the cervix. As with the cervical cap, spermicide is applied before insertion. The diaphragm achieved widespread use amongst upper-middle-class women in the decades immediately prior to the introduction of intrauterine devices (IUDs) and the contraceptive pill. Medical problems associated with its use are extremely uncommon apart from rare allergic reactions to the latex or spermicide; the two main problems are those of proper fit and/or proper use. Vaginal barriers such as the diaphragm require professional advice for selection of the size and training in fitting.

The first female condom (Figure 8.5) was launched in 1988, and the packaging process of femidom® is shown in Figure 8.6. A female condom under the trade-name Reality® is available in the United States. It is a prelubricated sheath, but, instead of covering the penis like an ordinary condom, it gently lines the vagina. It is inserted in a similar way to a tampon and is held in place at the upper end of the vagina by a small ring inside the sheath (Figure 8.7). This does not require precise placement over the cervix. A ring at the open end lies against the vulva during intercourse, preventing the whole sheath from slipping inside. Like the more traditional male equivalent, the female condom protects against pregnancy and provides a barrier to HIV and other sexually transmissible organisms.

This device is the first widely available condom to be made of polyurethane: a stronger material than latex which, however, is soft and comfortable, allowing a greater degree of sensitivity for many couples. The lubricant used is non-spermicidal silicone fluid. Clinical studies have revealed no serious safety issues and there are no reports of allergy to polyurethane or the lubricant. The impermeability of the condom to various sexually transmissible organisms has been demonstrated, and the contraceptive efficacy has been shown to be the same as those of other female-controlled barrier methods. As with any type of barrier contraceptive, it may take a little practice for the couple to become accustomed to the condom and adept at using it. Each female condom must be used only once.

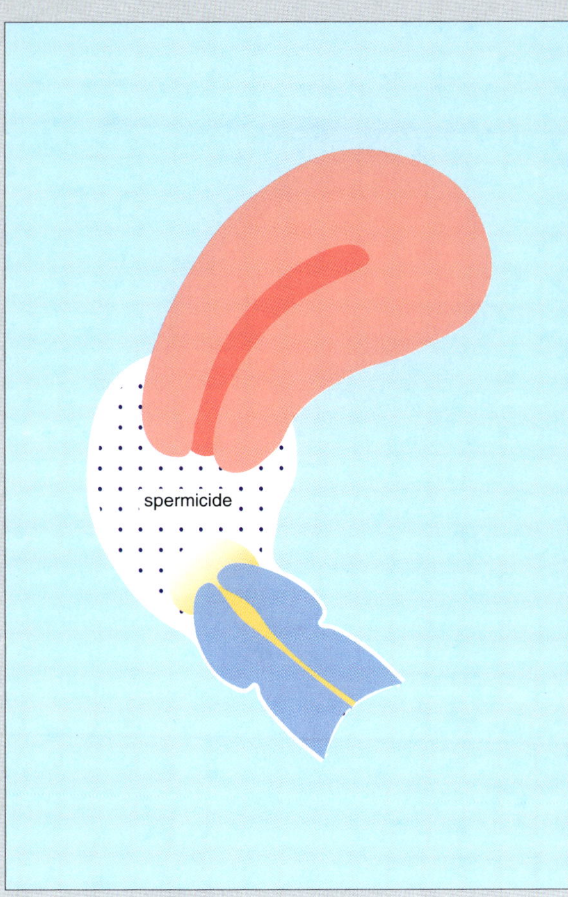

Figure 8.1 Site of action of spermicides which can be used alone or in combination with a barrier

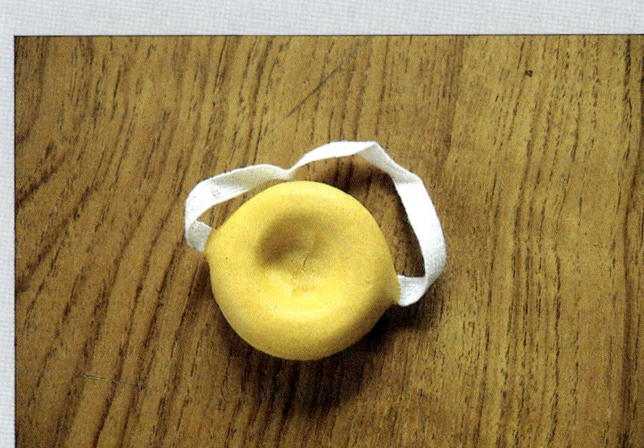

Figure 8.2 Disposable plastic sponge

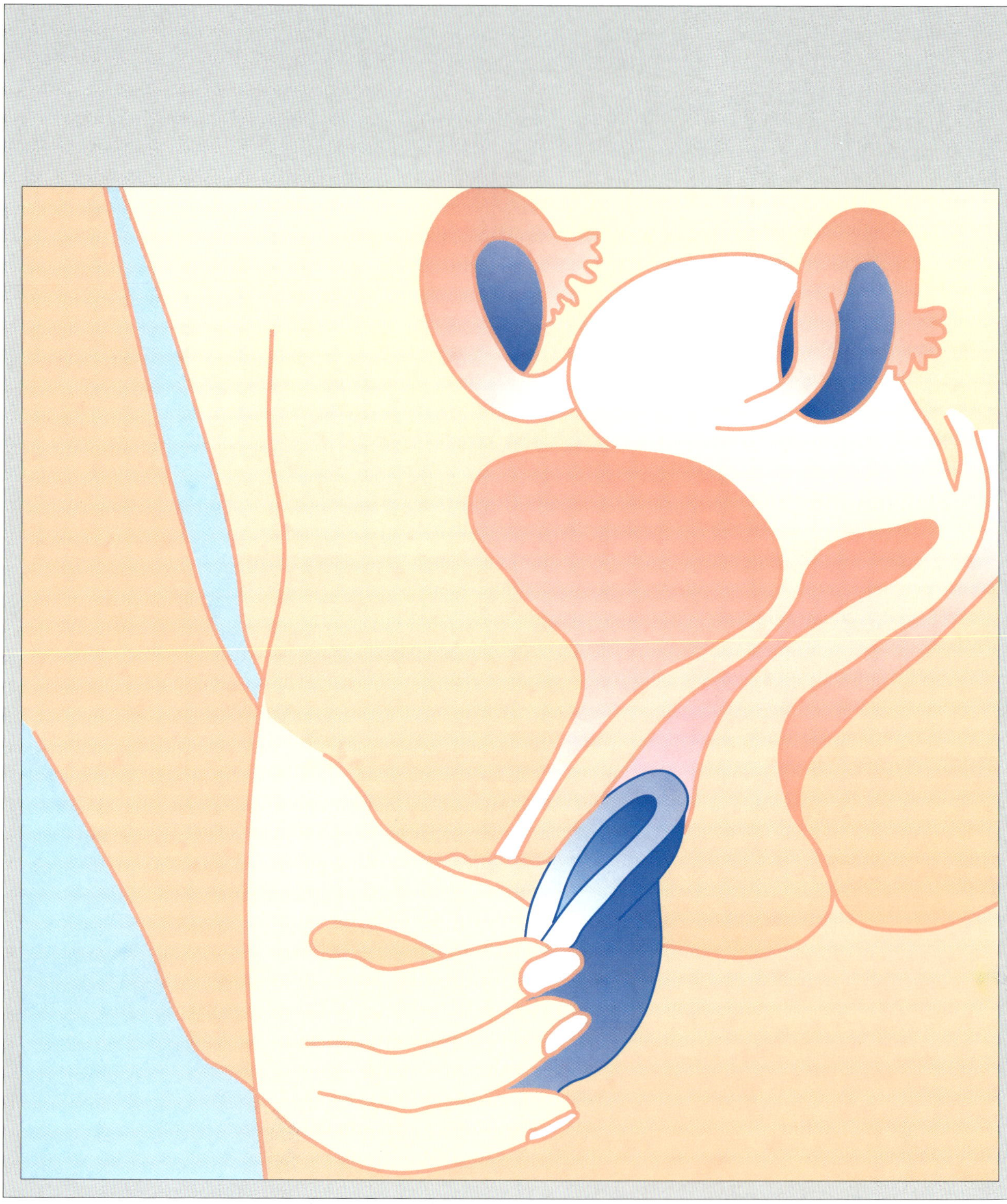

Figure 8.3 Cross-sectional view of the correct positioning of the diaphragm. (Adapted from Stoppard, M. (1983). *Every Woman's Life Guide*, p. 183. (London: McDonald & Co.))

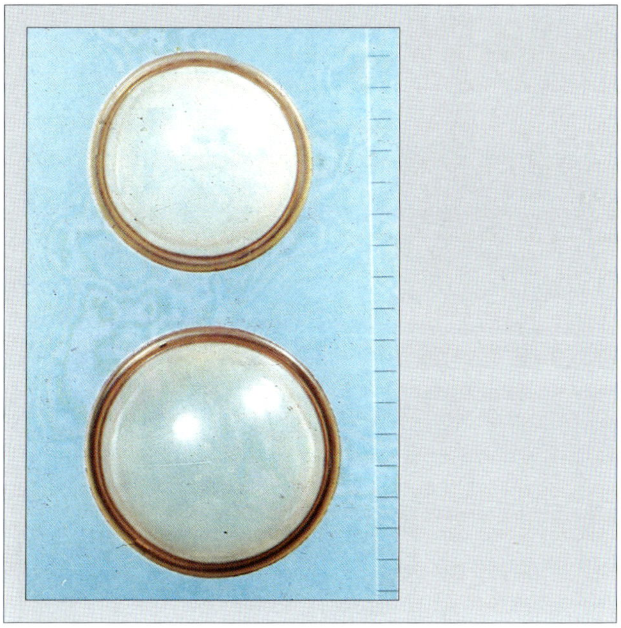

Figure 8.4 Two examples of the diaphragm

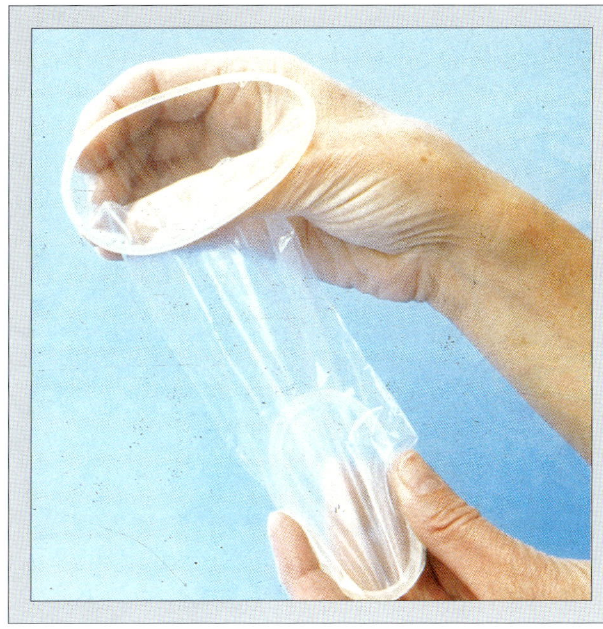

Figure 8.5 The female condom

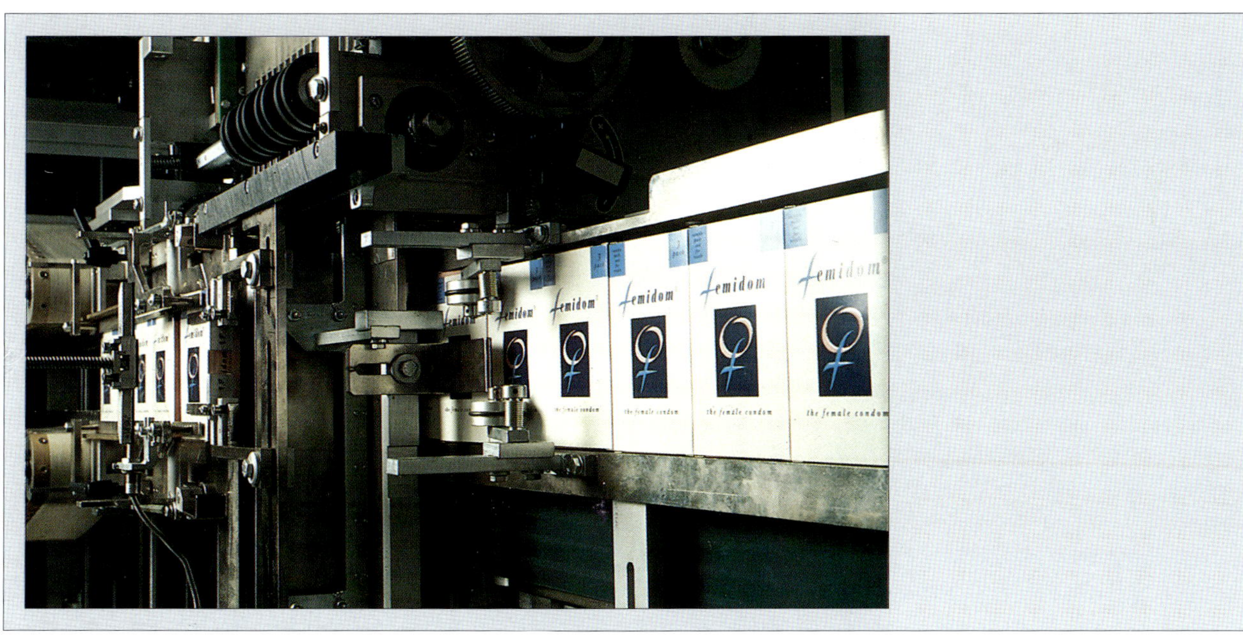

Figure 8.6 'Packaging' of the female condom, *femidom*®. (Reproduced with kind permission from Chartex International PLC, London, UK)

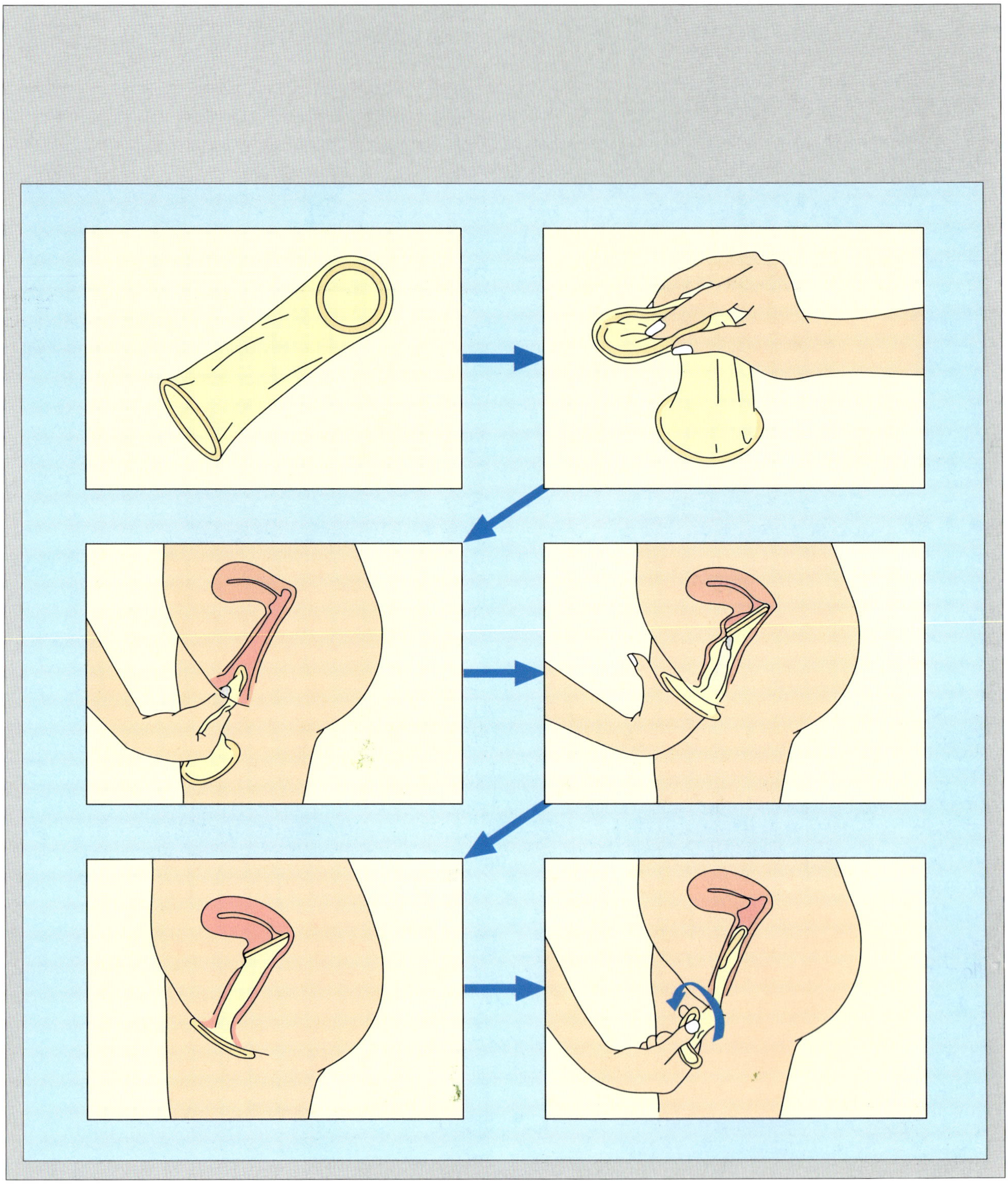

Figure 8.7 Insertion of the female condom, *femidom*®. (Reproduced with kind permission from Chartex International PLC, London, UK)

9

Intrauterine devices

As the need for fertility control grew at the end of the nineteenth century, important innovations in contraception occurred. The first was the development of the intrauterine device (IUD). IUDs were derived from stem pessaries, which were conceived as devices rather like over-large drawing pins (thumb tacks) designed to prevent the ascent of sperm through the cervix (Figure 9.1). In order to hold them in place, a Y-shaped metal extension was inserted in the uterus. It was observed that, even when the cervical device broke off, the intrauterine metallic portion still exerted a contraceptive effect.

Even to this day there is some dispute over how IUDs work; their effect may be through a number of complementary mechanisms which include changing the uterine environment in order to make implantation of the fertilized egg impossible, as well as reducing the number and motility of sperm reaching the Fallopian tubes and perhaps bringing about changes in tubal physiology; ovum transport and embryo formation may also be affected. The main clinical advantages and disadvantages of IUDs were well understood by the first decade of the twentieth century. The devices were widely used by Gräfenberg and others in Europe between the two World Wars. As with many methods of contraception, they can be wonderfully effective (98%) and acceptable, but they also have important limitations and strong contraindications.

An IUD gives long-term, easily reversible, coitally independent contraceptive protection; it does not require continuous motivation for effective use. IUDs are associated with heavier menstruation, although with the new generation of copper and hormonal devices this has been largely overcome. IUDs must be inserted and removed by trained health workers under strict aseptic conditions. Possible side-effects include pain, increased bleeding, infection and contraceptive failure. Perforation is possible and is marginally more common postpartum and after second-trimester abortion when the uterus is soft or during lactation when the uterus can be very small. IUDs can be inserted any time in the menstrual cycle and special techniques are available for immediate (within 30 min) insertion after the delivery of the placenta. The failure rate of the new copper-bearing device can be less than two in 100 woman-years of exposure.

The main disadvantage of IUDs is that they increase the relative risk of genital infections. They should not be used in women who have multiple sexual partners or whose partners have multiple partners. They are rarely appropriate for women who have never had any children. Contraindications include acute or chronic pelvic inflammatory disease, known or suspected pregnancy, abnormal uterine bleeding, malignancy of the genital tract and abnormalities of the uterine cavity. Figure 9.2 shows the mortality from IUDs compared with other reversible methods and no birth control.

Figure 9.3 shows several types of IUD, and Figure 9.4 illustrates the insertion of one such device.

By a sad quirk of history, major improvements in IUDs (in particular the addition of copper to flexible plastic T-shaped devices, which led to lower pregnancy rates with less menstrual disturbances), together with a good epidemiological understanding of the contraindications, occurred at the very time that the A. H. Robins Company made major and serious mistakes with the Dalkon Shield (see Figure 9.3). It is characteristic of nearly all methods of contraception that their acceptability and pregnancy rates are reported to be lowest in carefully supervised clinical trials. In the case of the Dalkon Shield, some of the early users also inserted spermicides around the time of ovulation and the published failure rates were unrealistically low, although this double protection was not explicitly mentioned in relevant publications. Cases of serious pelvic infection occurred with the Dalkon Shield, and some women who became pregnant with the device in place became seriously ill. A. H. Robins had been bankrupted as a result; more importantly, from the point of view of health of women, unreasonable suspicion and pessimism have fallen on all other IUDs, which are less widely used in the Western world than experience would otherwise justify. IUDs remain the most common single method of contraception in the People's Republic of China. Globally, 60 million women use them; of these, only 1.4 million are used by USA women and 600 000 in the UK.

Evidence indicates that effective postcoital contraception can be achieved by the insertion of a copper-containing IUD (Figure 9.4) within 5 days of unprotected sexual intercourse. This method may be used when there is a need for continuing contraception and/or where there is a contraindication for use of the pill postcoitally. Special care should be taken when providing IUDs postcoitally, especially if the client is at risk of pelvic inflammatory disease.

Two of the more frequent side-effects of the more widely used IUDs are bleeding and pain. By careful screening of clients, empathetic client counseling and proper care in IUD insertion, the incidence of these side-effects has been reduced. However, discontinuation rates for their complaints remain high.

LEVONORGESTREL IUD

The levonorgestrel-releasing IUD combines the positive characteristics of oral contraceptives, IUDs and steroid-releasing implants. It is particularly attractive to women suffering from menorrhagia and dysmenorrhea. Levo-Nova®, registered in Finland, has a daily release of 20 μg levonorgestrel and an estimated effective life of up to 7 years.

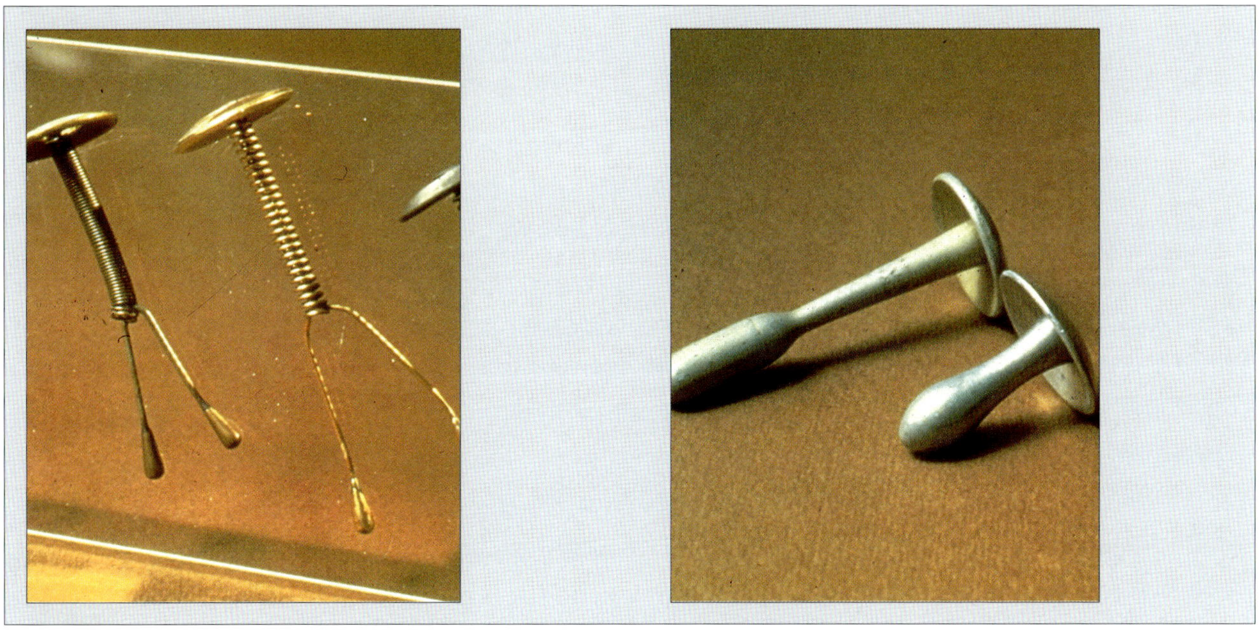

Figure 9.1 Early IUDs. Forerunners of the intrauterine device were the intracervical stems (right) and wishbone intracervical device (left). The stems were sutured to the uterine wall via the small hole in the rim. The wishbone devices were placed in the cervix and the stem protruded into the uterus. (Reproduced with kind permission from the Ortho-McNeil Inc., Canada)

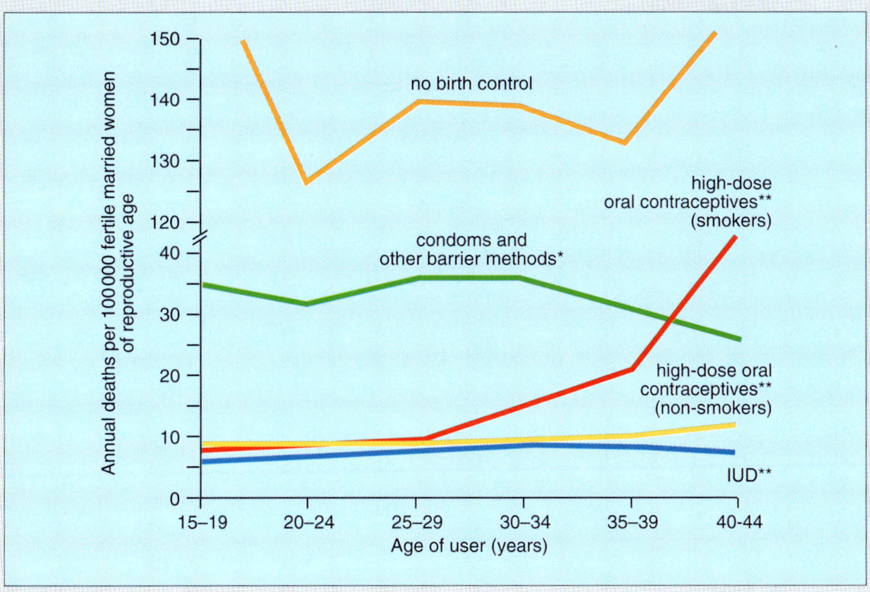

Figure 9.2 Mortality from intrauterine devices compared with other reversible methods and no birth control. Estimated annual deaths resulting from pregnancy, childbirth, contraceptive use, and unintended pregnancy following contraceptive failure, by age of women in low-income developing countries. *, Pregnancy-related deaths; **, method and pregnancy-related deaths. (Adapted from Sciarra, J.J. *et al.* (1978). *Risks, Benefits and Controversies in Fertility Control.* (Hagerstown, Maryland: Harker & Row))

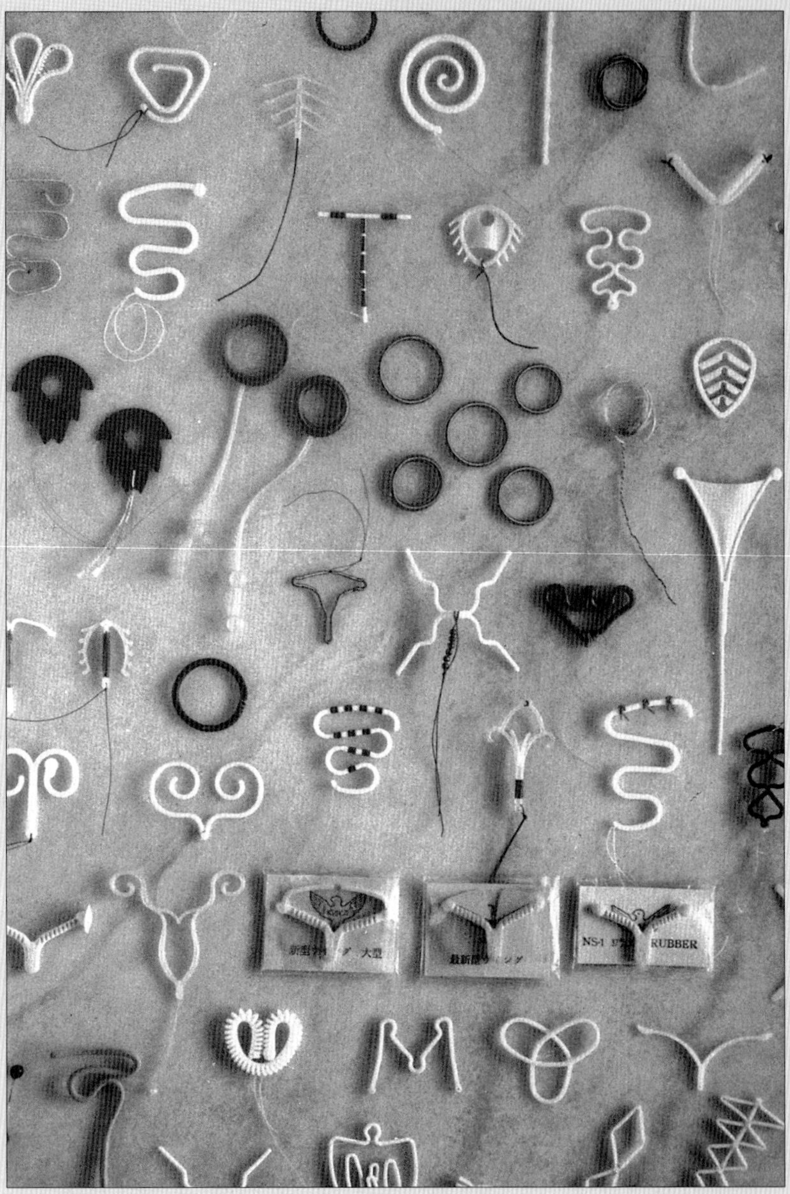

Figure 9.3 An assortment of intrauterine devices

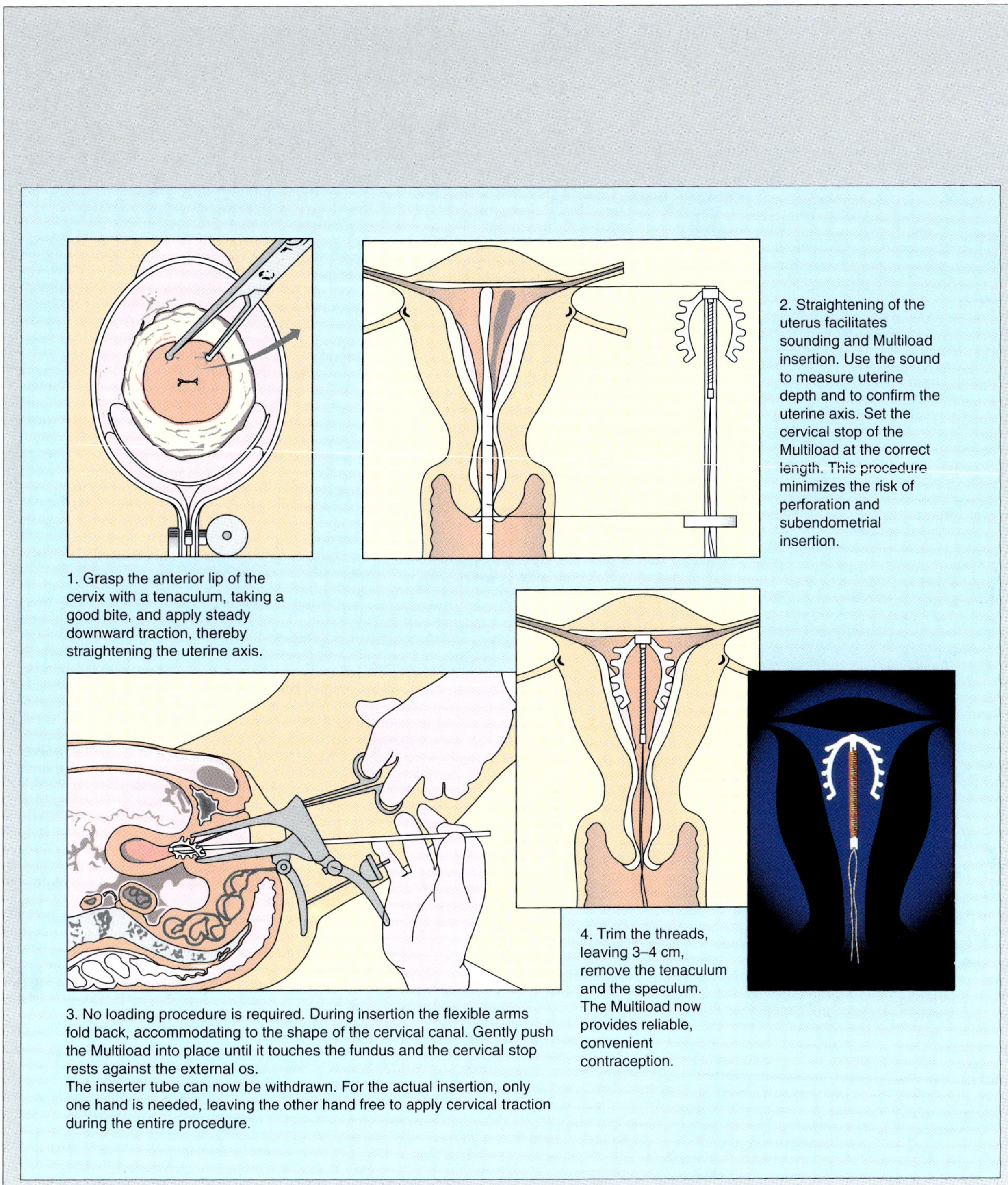

Figure 9.4 The insertion of one type of intrauterine device

10

Periodic abstinence and coitus interruptus

Until the early twentieth century it was believed that women were maximally fertile at the time of menstruation. In the 1930s Ogino and Knaus demonstrated that ovulation occurs 14 days before the next menstrual period, and soon efforts were made to develop a method of family planning using this information. The rhythm or calendar method is based on predicting the time of ovulation solely on the basis of the length of previous cycles.

One of the effects of estrogen is alteration of the cervical mucus from a thick, opaque sticky consistency to a thin, clear lubricant substance close to the time of ovulation. Progesterone produces a rise in basal body temperature after ovulation. In the basal body temperature method, the woman records her temperature on waking each morning to establish the basal reading; a rise of 0.2–0.4 °C occurs at ovulation and the higher reading persists until the onset of menstruation (Figure 10.1). Because of the limited life of the ovum (it can be fertilized for only about 12 h after release), the woman waits until 3 consecutive days of recording at the higher temperature and can then start intercourse with little risk of conception. Because sperm can survive for up to 3 days, intercourse must be avoided in the first part of the cycle between menstruation and ovulation (the basal body temperature method cannot predict ovulation), although for part of that time the woman will be infertile. This method requires a long time of abstinence in each cycle but has a high degree of reliability, the rate of unexpected pregnancies varying from less than one to about 6/100 woman-years of use. It is not, however, a practical method for women with very irregular cycles.

The cervical mucus method involves observation, both by sensation and visual inspection, of the texture of mucus which appears at the vulva. There may be a number of 'dry days' following menstruation; thereafter, with rising estrogen levels, the mucus becomes thick and sticky and then progressively thin, clear and slippery until the 'peak' day, after which it again changes. Abstinence is necessary from the time the mucus appears until the 4th day after peak, when intercourse can be resumed and continued as often as desired until the next menstrual period. The duration of abstinence is shorter by this method than by the basal body temperature technique; however, the frequency of unexpected pregnancies is higher, from five to 35/100 woman-years. A 'symptothermal' method combines these two methods of periodic abstinence, and wide variations in the pregnancy rate have been reported – from four to 26 per 100 woman-years. Ovulation methods need to be carefully tested, but once a couple have learnt the techniques of ovulation prediction, and have the motivation and discipline to practice abstinence when required, no further inputs are needed. Unintended pregnancies, however, sometimes occur during the learning phase.

The identification of the fertile phase can be combined with the use of a barrier method only during those days estimated to be the fertile phase of the woman's cycle (Figure 10.2). Recognition of the time of ovulation is also useful for women seeking to become pregnant, especially if some degree of infertility exists. Self-palpation of the cervix, which softens as ovulation approaches, is another method of timing of periodic abstinence; however, its efficacy has not yet been determined.

Many family planning clients find periodic abstinence more difficult to use than many other methods. Nevertheless, it is better than no method at all, and may be the only choice for some individuals and couples. Interestingly, Saint Augustine condemned the use of what today we would call the rhythm or periodic abstinence method of family planning; despite the early condemnation by theologians, the method has become the only one formally approved in recent Papal encyclicals.

COITUS INTERRUPTUS

The practice of contraception is one of the factors that distinguishes us from other animals: chimpanzees use tools, albeit simple ones, and can be taught a sign language, but, as an Islamic theologian observed long ago, we are the only animal that consciously controls our fertility. Perhaps, instead of calling ourselves *Homo sapiens* (the 'wise' man), we should call ourselves *Homo contraceptus*. As noted, coitus interruptus not only has an ancient lineage, but its simplicity and anonymity made it the commonest method of family planning throughout much of Western Europe and the rest of the world. Advantages include the fact that this method is always available, at no cost! but the failure rate is high, and withdrawal may not always be in time! (Figure 10.3). The data that are available on failure rates suggest they overlap with those of condoms and mechanical methods. As long ago as the sixteenth century, Saint Bernadine of Sienna wrote, 'Of one thousand marriages I believe 990 are the devils', that is, were using coitus interruptus.

As part of the medicalization of fertility regulation, coitus interruptus has come in for some fanciful criticisms, including the possibility of physical and psychological damage. The reality is that human sexual behavior is highly malleable and if a couple love one another they can express that love through coitus interruptus. Coitus interruptus may have become widespread in the West as a result of the criticism of the Church and explicit questions which have been asked for hundreds of years in the confessional. To the ancient Jews and early Christians, semen was a perfect whole and the male was thought to plant his 'seed' in the female, who was not understood to make any contribution to the next generation. By the time of the Prophet Mohammed, the anatomy and physiology of the ovaries were beginning to be understood and it was appreciated that women made a contribution to procreation; and therefore, semen became incomplete. Masturbation and coitus interruptus became less reprehensible. In some contemporary countries, such as Turkey, coitus interruptus remains the major method of contraception and is becoming increasingly common as fertility declines. The often-quoted criticism that pre-ejaculatory fluid contains sperm which might lead to accidental fertilization has no grounds in reproductive physiology – if such a small number of sperm were found in the ejaculate of a man seeking treatment for infertility, he would be considered an incurable case. Coitus interruptus may give partial protection against transmitting HIV disease.

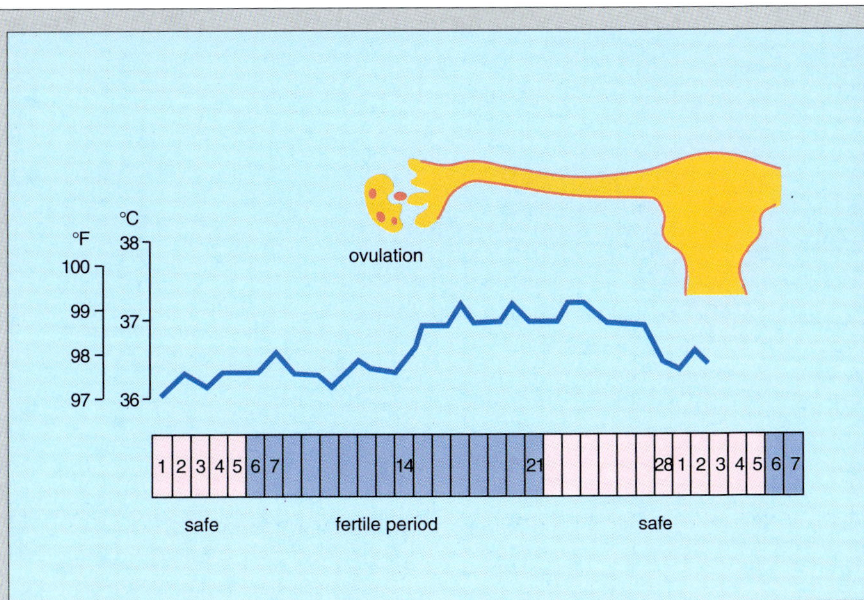

Figure 10.1 The basal body temperature method of periodic abstinence uses temperature recordings throughout the menstrual cycle; a rise of 0.2–0.4 °C occurs at ovulation and persists until the onset of menstruation

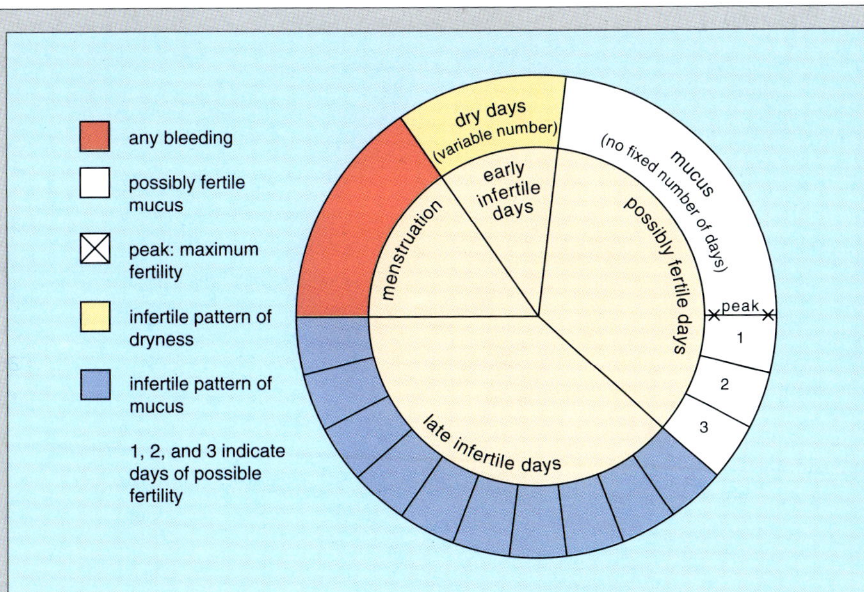

Figure 10.2 The mucus pattern of fertility and infertility during the menstrual cycle (peak indicates maximum fertility)

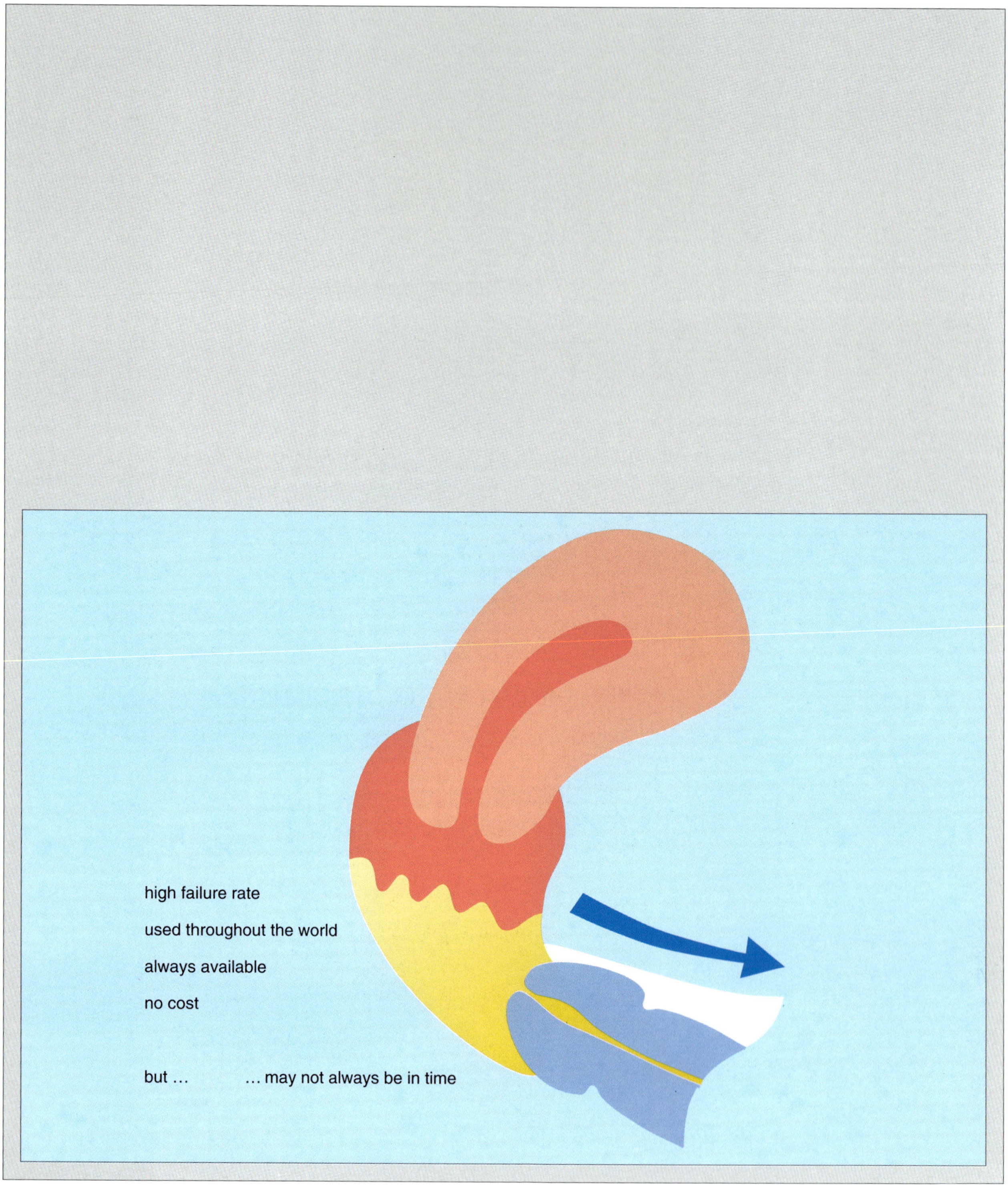

Figure 10.3 Coitus interruptus

11

Voluntary surgical contraception

In Britain and the USA, voluntary surgical contraception is the single most common modality of family planning. The reality is that even though there is now a good choice of satisfactory modern methods of contraception, failure of the methods and, more importantly, human errors in use, are sufficiently common that over a fertile lifetime a very significant number of couples will have one or more unwanted pregnancies. Any community which is striving to have a small family size must either accept the limitations of reversible methods and be prepared to back them up with safe abortion, or offer a choice of voluntary surgical contraception. Wherever this choice has been made available, it has become an increasingly important part of the family planning choices.

Voluntary surgical contraception is common in a number of developing countries where fertility has declined rapidly, such as Thailand and Colombia. Where it has been available for several decades, as in the USA, Korea or Britain, both male and female operations are performed in large numbers. It is common, however, for female sterilization to be offered before male, often beginning with women who have genuine medical contraindications to additional pregnancies, such as diabetes. Female sterilization also makes particular sense to women who have so much more to invest in pregnancy and bringing up children than men, as well as the fact that sterilization in some ways merely represents bringing the infertility aspect of the menopause forward by some years.

Voluntary surgical contraception appears to be attractive to many people in a variety of cultures. Where it is poorly used it is not stopped so much by lack of need, as by a lack of a medical tradition to make the operation available. When programs first make voluntary surgical contraception available, they often apply arbitrary rules of age and parity for client eligibility (e.g. the woman's age and number of children multiplied together should equal 120). With the passage of time these criteria are nearly always abandoned and sterilization becomes a choice which is made available to individuals who understand the nature of the operation and are clear they do not want any more children.

Candidates for voluntary surgical contraception include:

(1) Those who have completed their families;

(2) Those who don't want children;

(3) Women with a poor obstetric history; and

(4) Those with genetic reasons for not having children.

Sterilization, male or female, is usually the most effective method of contraception. It is a one-time procedure which is relatively simple in either sex. It does not require constant use of a method or a check-up at regular intervals or the cost of contraceptive supplies. The risk of complications is minimal if the procedure is performed to strict medical standards. Sterilization operations usually demand a greater degree of skill, training and equipment than temporary methods of contraception. However, they often also give many years of complete protection against pregnancy and are therefore generally more cost-effective than such reversible methods. Figure 11.1 outlines the advantages and disadvantages of surgical sterilization.

LEGAL AND ETHICAL ISSUES

The use of sterilization has been constrained by statute law in two ways: often it has been forbidden, or over-regulated, and in a few cases – fortunately more talked about than implemented – the state has tried to make sterilization compulsory under certain circumstances.

Sterilization was never illegal in Britain, although vasectomy did not become part of comprehensive services until 1979. In the USA, some states passed coercive sterilization laws in the first half of this century, although they have now all been repealed. In 1976, the State of Marharastra in India passed a law imposing fines and imprisonment on anyone with three or more children who refused to be sterilized. The law, however, was never ratified before Mrs Gandhi's government fell.

Some countries, such as Bangladesh, give a small monetary compensation or 'incentive' for male or female sterilization. Incidentally, no one in India has ever received a transistor radio for a vasectomy – it was suggested by an enthusiastic administrator but was never put into practice.

VASECTOMY

Vasectomy (male sterilization) has had a chequered history, beginning in the 1920s with charlatans who claimed that vasectomy led to male rejuvenation. The operation that is usually practiced today was perfected in India in the 1950s. It is a simple 5-minute procedure performed under a local anesthetic during which the vas deferens is isolated, ligated and the two ends tied or the lumen cauterized (Figures 11.2–11.5). The key to success is for the surgeon to identify and fix the vas with his fingers prior to surgery. The operation can even be done through a single, tiny incision using a sharp forceps – the 'no-scalpel' vasectomy which has now entered widespread use. It was developed by Dr Li Shungiang in China. As in routine vasectomy the vas is palpated below the skin of the scrotum. The skin is then perforated with a special pair of forceps. The vas is extracted and occluded. The method is slightly more difficult to learn but is associated with less bleeding and the puncture wound in the skin is so slight that no suture is needed.

Possible complications of vasectomy include: vasovagal attack, pain, bleeding with hematoma, infection, sinus formation, sperm granuloma and failure, and psychological sequelae. Vasectomy is not immediately effective. The client has to use condoms or his partner another temporary method until he has had 15–30 ejaculations after vasectomy or until sperm-free semen is demonstrated using semen analysis.

Vasectomy is not recommended as the best method of contraception if the man has a history of impotence or if he has a psychological fear of the procedure or its consequences; or if the wife requires hysterectomy for any reason; or if the marriage faces problems.

FEMALE STERILIZATION

Female sterilization, which requires tubal occlusion using one of a variety of techniques including surgery, electrocautery and the application of clips and rings, necessitates opening the abdominal cavity (Figure 11.6). It is always going to be a more complicated procedure than the male operation. Nevertheless, there have been some remarkable simplifications of technology in the last 20 years, particularly the use of the so-called minilaparotomy where the Fallopian tubes are occluded through an abdominal incision measuring 2–5 cm, and which is usually carried out using local anesthesia and light sedation. Sterilization can also be performed through a 2-cm incision under local anesthesia using a laparoscope to locate and occlude the tubes. It has been dubbed the 'band-aid' operation, and can be done on a day-care basis. A variety of mechanical clips, including the Filshie Clip™ (Figure 11.7) and rings have been devised which can be placed with a laparoscope. Clips do minimal damage to the Fallopian tube, making the possibility of repair more likely. Electric cautery can also be used but destroys much more of the Fallopian tube. Cautery has an even lower failure rate than clips or rings. Complications of minilaparotomy include those of the anesthetic, immediate surgical complications (trauma, hemorrhage), and delayed problems (hemorrhage, infection and failure).

Recently a further simplification to female sterilization, where the procedure does not involve surgery, has become available, with the use of quinacrine. The method, developed by Jaime Zipper in Chile, uses a small inserter (about the size of a drinking straw) to place pellets of quinacrine in the uterus (Figure 11.8). These dissolve and destroy the endometrium and the cells lining the Fallopian tubes. The endometrium regenerates after this 'chemical curettage', but the tubes become fibrosed. The method is simpler than having an IUD inserted: it does have a failure rate and must be repeated at least once. Among 32 000 quinacrine procedures in Vietnam, there were no recorded deaths, whereas over 200 maternal deaths would have occurred in this group of women without sterilization. Quinacrine has a failure rate of 2.6 pregnancies per 100 women after one year of exposure. The toxicology studies on the safety of quinacrine have not yet been fully established and this is preventing the wider use of this technique.

Tubal ligation significantly reduces the risk of ovarian cancer, as illustrated in Figure 11.9

Voluntary surgical contraception should be accepted only when a couple are clear that they want no more children. If disaster strikes, however, and children die prematurely or divorce occurs, then techniques for attempting to restore fertility exist. In the female they involve major operative surgery and, even when successful, carry an inevitable risk of a tubal instead of a uterine pregnancy. In the male, reversal is somewhat easier and does not carry any comparable risk; however, though patency of tubes can be achieved, fertility cannot always be guaranteed.

Female sterlization

- The effect is immediate, but there is no way of judging the effectiveness of the procedure
- Postoperative recovery is rapid (ambulatory after a few to 48 h) and a hospital stay of only 12–48 h as necessary
- The operation can be classified as an outpatient procedure
- The procedure can be performed under local anesthesia (minimal risk); if general anesthesia is necessary then the risks associated with this apply
- Reversal of the procedure is successful in up to 75% of cases, depending on the particular method of sterilization.
- However, there is a risk of ectopic pregnancy following reversal
- The operation provides an opportunity to explore the pelvic cavity for gynecological problems. However, there may be operative risk to other organs
- The risk of ovarian cancer is reduced

Vasectomy

- The operation is quick, easy and safe
- Two negative sperm counts assume sterility, but repeat visits for sperm counts are necessary, 15–30 postoperative ejaculations being needed before sterility occurs
- The operation can be classified as an outpatient procedure
- The procedure can be performed under local anesthesia which is associated with minimal risk
- Reversal of the procedure is easier as compared to that of female sterilization, provided that the reversal is carried out fairly soon after vasectomy

Figure 11.1 Voluntary surgical contraception: the advantages and disadvantages

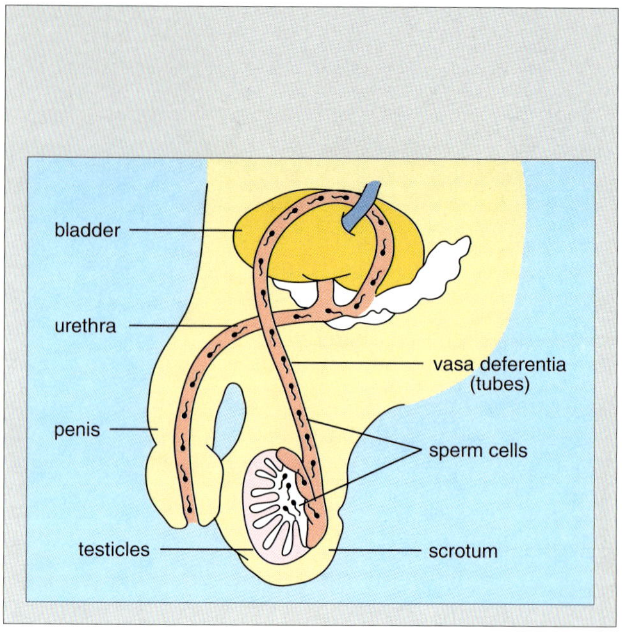

Figure 11.2 Lateral view of the male reproductive organs illustrating how the sperm pass freely through the male reproductive tract

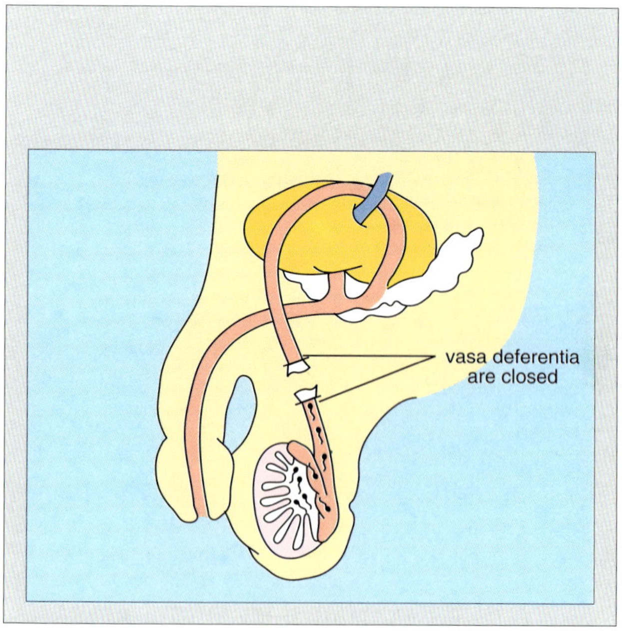

Figure 11.3 Lateral view of the male reproductive organs illustrating how, after vasectomy, the vasa deferentia are blocked, and sperm cells are prevented from reaching and joining female egg cells

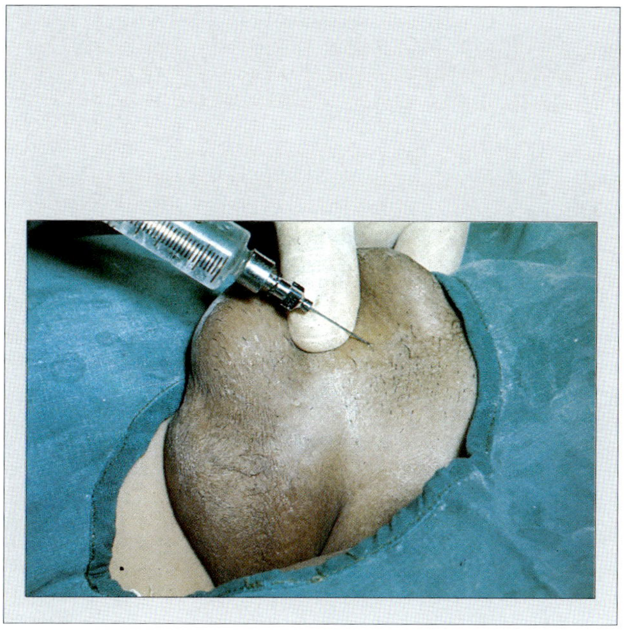

Figure 11.4 Modern vasectomy is a simple procedure which can be done under local anesthesia

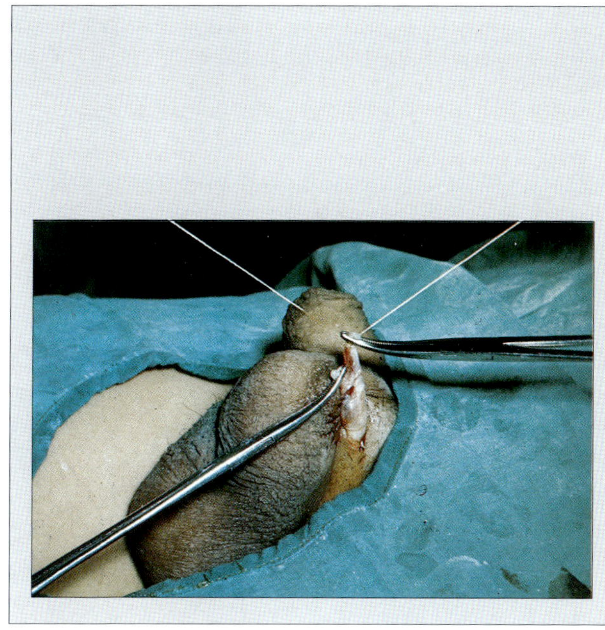

Figure 11.5 Vasectomy: the vas deferens is isolated and ligated

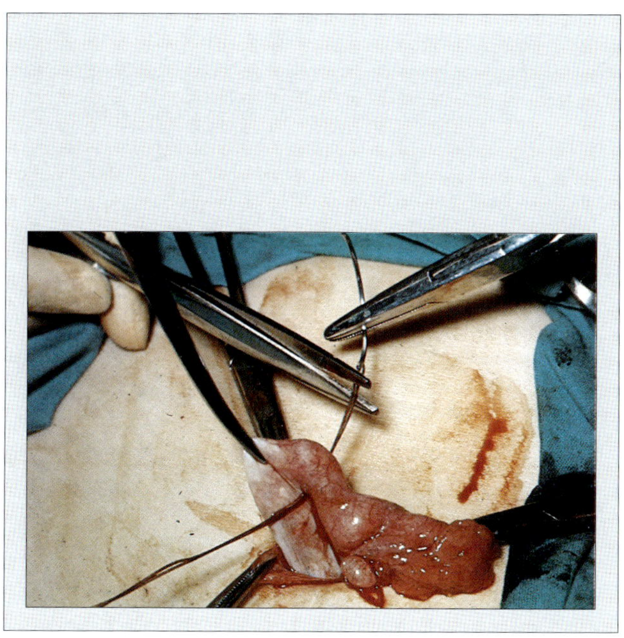

Figure 11.6 Female sterilization: the abdomen is opened through small incisions and the Fallopian tubes are isolated and occluded

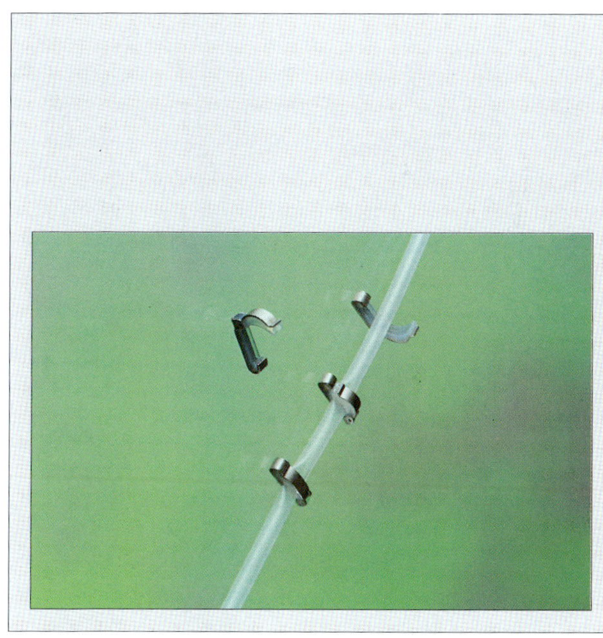

Figure 11.7 Filshie Clip™.(Reproduced with kind permission from Femcare Ltd., Nottingham, England)

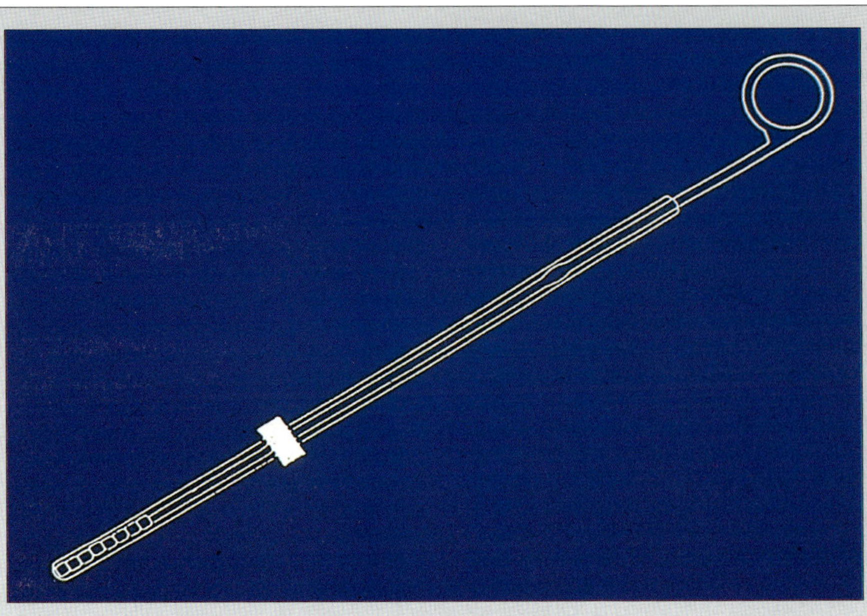

Figure 11.8 Quinacrine tablet inserter

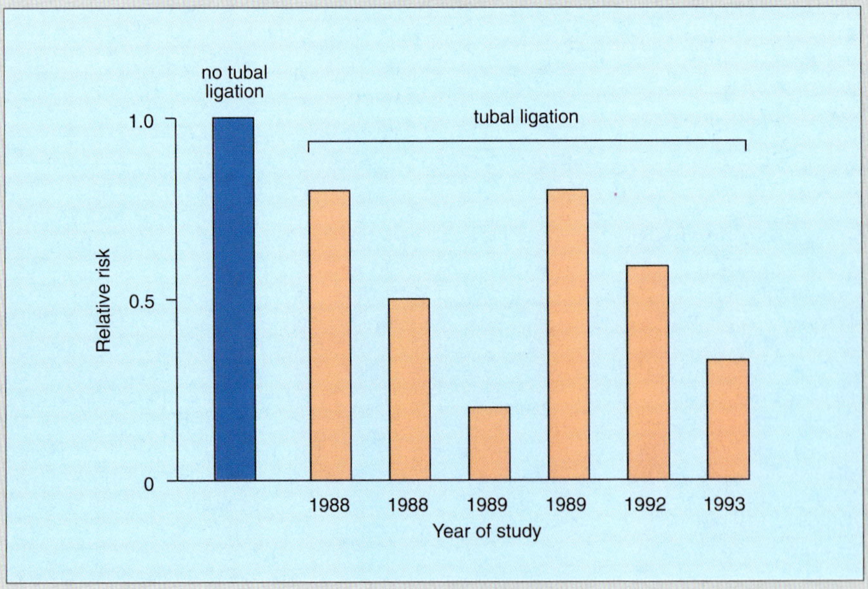

Figure 11.9 Relative risk of ovarian cancer after tubal ligation. (Data from Hankinson, S.E. *et al.* (1993). Tubal ligation, hysterectomy, and risk of ovarian cancer. *J. Am. Med. Assoc.*, **270**, 2816)

12

Contraception for special groups

All currently available methods of modern contraceptives are safe, effective and reliable. As such, they are suitable for most individuals. However, contraceptive needs differ for different groups of individuals, and also within groups, and differences occur among different individuals. For example, the contraceptive needs of the young unmarried girl will be different to those of a young married couple in a stable union. Again, the needs of the couple will vary, depending on whether they are delaying the first pregnancy or whether they need a method to space between pregnancies. The same couple's needs will change once their family is complete, when they would do better with a more permanent method. Just as contraceptive needs differ at different stages of one's reproductive life, similarly, specific groups of individuals can be identified who may have specific contraceptive needs. Though there are many such groups, four groups will be highlighted.

ADOLESCENTS

One of the outstanding features of fertility today is the very high pregnancy rates among married and unmarried women under 20 years of age in countries all over the world, both developing and developed. These high pregnancy rates constitute a major risk for the health and social wellbeing of the younger woman and her child (see Chapter 2, section on *Health Rationale*). It is, therefore, important to protect the young woman from unwanted pregnancy at this time.

In almost all countries of the world, the age of puberty is decreasing (Chapter 2) and yet girls are marrying later. Though physically mature, they are not considered socially mature and ready for marriage. This gap has been termed the 'biosocial gap' and is widening (Figure 12.1). In many countries the age of first intercourse is also falling. These factors result in increasing numbers of pregnancies to unmarried adolescents. In additon, in many traditional societies, girls are still entering into marriage at a young age. These factors contribute to a rise in the incidence of tubal pregnancies.

For the young adolescent, there are hazards to health associated with sexuality. For example, the tissues of the cervical epithelium seem more susceptible to dysplasia under the precipitating influence of one or several factors contributed to by the male. Relationships tend to be less stable, and if there is more than one partner involved, there will be the increased risk of sexually transmissible infections. Perhaps the most complex in its consequences, however, is the birth of children to inexperienced and immature mothers. This situation is made worse when there is inadequate social support.

Reproductive Health clinics serving young people should provide an attractive and informal setting, staffed by well-trained and caring people who are not likely to prejudge the moral issues or adversely stereotype their clients. Ideally, counseling should be available for young people of either sex.

No single method of contraception can be considered suitable for adolescents as a group, but factors such as age, parity, sexual habits, risks of infection, risks of pregnancy, etc. should be considered prior to providing a method. Oral contraceptives may be prescribed for adolescents although caution is recommended in prescribing for very young girls. Other methods of contraception are to be preferred until regular menstruation is established. However, if sexually active adolescents are not able to use other methods, then the pill may be prescribed since the social, medical and psychological consequences of pregnancy and abortion outweigh any physiological reservations that may exist.

Other hormonal methods such as injectables can be used, and NORPLANT® can be used in older adolescents. They should not be considered methods of first choice for this age group, particularly nulliparous adolescents.

Intrauterine devices are not the method of first choice for nulliparous women or a woman who is likely to have more than one partner.

Barrier methods, including diaphragms and condoms (male and female), are good methods of contraception for highly motivated adolescents who are able to use these methods consistently and correctly.

Spermicides, when used with diaphragms or condoms, ensure high effectiveness. Used alone, they are less effective; but these methods are usually easy to obtain and use, and this may be an advantage, particularly for adolescents. They may have a protective effect over some sexually transmissible diseases and pelvic inflammatory disease. Withdrawal and periodic abstinence are not reliable methods, particularly for the adolescent. In adolescents, sexual control may be low, leading to higher failure rates with coitus interruptus. Periodic abstinence relies on attempts to identify the time of ovulation and this is dependent on regular cycles. This method is also difficult to use by those who only have occasional sexual intercourse.

Sterilization is rarely indicated in this age group and should be considered only in exceptional medically dictated circumstances.

CONTRACEPTION FOR THE OLDER WOMAN

For women over 35 years of age (regarded obstetrically as 'older women') there are particular needs and problems associated with contraception. The ability to conceive continues to decrease with age until the menopause. So these women, on the one hand, may not need very effective methods of contraception. However, on the other hand, an accidental pregnancy for a woman in her forties may be a very traumatic experience. So a balance has to be struck. Women in this age group may be more prone to conditions such as obesity, hypertension and diabetes which, together with smoking, are risk factors for adverse cardiovascular effects when taking oral contraceptives. Figure 12.2 illustrates the relationship between estrogen and progesterone dosage of combined oral contraceptives and the incidence of total arterial disease. At the lowest dosage of estrogen and progesterone, no deaths were seen.

The risk of developing cardiovascular and other diseases appears to be greater among women who take pills with higher doses of estrogen and more potent progestins. There is virtually no reason for a woman to take an oral contraceptive that contains more than 50 μg of estrogen. Yet, more than one million USA women – about 12% of all pill users – do so (Figure 12.3). What is more, older pill users – those at highest risk – are over five times more likely to be taking a high-dose pill than those in the youngest age group. To minimize risk, it is advisable that women currently taking high-dose pills switch to a preparation containing 50 μg or less of estrogen, and that women commencing pill use start with a low-dose pill.

Sterilization is a suitable option for many women over 35, and female sterilization or vasectomy is being selected increasingly by couples of this age group whose family size is complete. Both procedures have very low rates of failure and the simple operation can be carried out under local anesthetic.

Combined oral contraceptives can be used for the older woman who has no risk factor for cardiovascular complications. Even women over 40 who have no risk factors can still consider using the pill with appropriate information. The progestogen-only pill, on the other hand, is suitable for women until menopause.

Other hormonal methods such as injectables or implants can be useful for the older woman. There is at present no evidence of adverse medical effects enhanced by age with these methods.

Intrauterine devices are another method suitable for older women. Menstrual loss can be increased and women should be warned, particularly at this age, about this side-effect. Devices should be removed about a year before menopause (although some can be recovered up to 1 year after), otherwise cervical stenosis may make removal difficult or impossible without general anesthesia.

Barrier methods are often found acceptable to older women, and may be suitable, particularly since fertility at this age is reduced and pregnancy rates are low.

CONTRACEPTION FOR NURSING MOTHERS

The choice of method of contraception for breastfeeding mothers is important because the chosen methods, in addition to providing effective contraception, must not adversely affect the quantity and quality of breast milk or the health of the infant. The method, and when to start the method, are both important considerations.

There are no universal rules in determining when a breastfeeding woman should start a particular contraceptive method. The best solution may be the formation of a decision tree adapted to a woman's specific situation. An example of this is shown in Figure 12.4.

For a woman who is fully breastfeeding on demand, it is extremely unlikely that she will conceive at least for the first 6 months. Although the childspacing effect is most reliable during exclusive breastfeeding and during the first 6 months, many women who breastfeed fully or almost fully for longer periods have been protected against pregnancy considerably beyond 6 months. In countries where the duration of breastfeeding is long – a median duration of 19 months in Senegal or 31 months in Bangladesh, for example – breastfeeding contributes greatly to delaying conception. It is important to remember that the effect of breastfeeding on fertility is significant primarily during the period before menses return (Figure 12.6).

There are clear differences between the rates of ovulation and of pregnancy during lactational amenorrhea. Ovulation is a prerequisite for pregnancy, but the probability of conception during a single normal cycle is only 25%. Thus, even when progesterone production is adequate, the estimated pregnancy rates during amenorrhea would be very low (3.5 and 9.4 per 100 women at 6 and 12 months, respectively).

The probabilities of pregnancy are similar for studies in Chile and the pooled data collected by Family Health International, with the exception of the 12-month pregnancy rate observed in Chile, where a few breastfeeding women remain amenorrheic for a full year (Figure 12.7). If the mother decides to breastfeed, then she should be supported to carry out the decision. Support, for example, in the form of good nutrition, maternity leave and assistance with how to breastfeed should be made available. The option for these mothers to rely on the contraceptive effects of lactation should be carefully explained. Provided the mother understands and accepts the possibility of an unexpected early conception (2% of mothers will conceive before menses has resumed and if they are feeding on demand), some of them will find it convenient to breastfeed without the risks and inconvenience of another method of contraception. Most methods of contraception can be used during lactation, but particular attention is required in relation to hormonal methods.

Combined estrogen–progestogen pills are known to reduce milk volume. Therefore, it is best to avoid using a combined pill during lactation. If it is necessary to use a combined pill, it is best to use as low a dose as possible, and only after breastfeeding is well established.

If a hormonal method is to be used during lactation, progestogen-only preparations have the advantage that they appear to have little or no adverse effects on milk production (quality and volume). Injectables, implants or pills containing progestogen only can be used.

In general, the lowest effective dose of progestogen-only contraceptives is to be preferred to combined oral contraceptives during lactation. However, there is much to be said in favor of non-hormonal methods for breastfeeding mothers, because of the presence of very small amounts of hormone in the milk. Intrauterine devices, barrier methods and spermicides can also be used effectively during lactation.

Postpartum female sterilization is a simple procedure and is commonly performed under local anesthesia. If sterilization is performed immediately after delivery, there is no effect on milk output, but if the operation is carried out after 7–14 days, the procedure is associated with a sharp drop in milk volume. Alternatively, sterilization can be delayed until 6 weeks postpartum when the uterus has involuted and laparoscopic or minilaparotomy sterilization can be performed. Counseling is important prior to providing any method of contraception. In particular, adequate counseling is vital when postpartum procedures are carried out since the mother may not be in a state of mind to give full informed consent, and also because her decision may have to be based following full assessment of the health status of the newborn infant.

CONTRACEPTION FOR PERSONS WITH DISABILITIES

Attitudes towards the personal and sexual needs of the disabled are changing, not least among the disabled themselves.

When considering contraceptive needs of the disabled, it should be kept in mind that the disability could be physical or mental or both. Most disabled people want to lead as normal a life as possible and that may mean getting married and having children.

When considering those with physical disabilities, contraception may be unnecessary only for those whose handicap also affects sexual function, particularly for men who may not be able to sustain an erection and/or who may be infertile (for example, in spinal cord injury, spina bifida, and advanced stages of multiple sclerosis).

Women suffering from some disorders may be able to become pregnant. The choice of contraceptive will have to be decided by considering primarily the woman's needs with regard to whether she wants to get pregnant or not.

If she wants to postpone pregnancy or not get pregnant at all, the choice of method would once again depend very much on her disability, her partner's support and also on the type of method that she could use on a continuing basis.

With mental disability, there are further problems. These relate to the mental status, the ability to give informed consent, the problems that the individual might encounter with a pregnancy, for example, carrying a pregnancy to term, caring for a child. While details of specific methods of contraception for the disabled cannot be prescribed in a general fashion in a book such as this, suffice to alert the reader to the fact that the disabled person has rights similar to those enjoyed by 'normal' individuals and that those caring for the disabled should consider the sexuality of the disabled with regard to the provision of health care and family planning services.

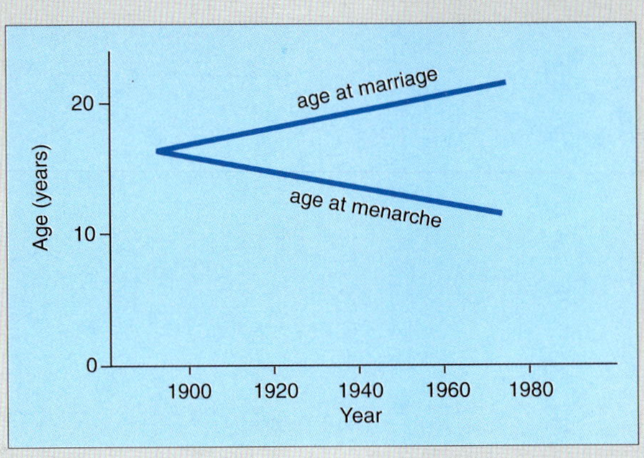

Figure 12.1 The 'biosocial gap' – the gap between age at marriage and age at menarche, 1900–1980. (Adapted from Rosenfield, A. and Fathalla, M. F. (1990). *The Figo Manual of Human Reproduction, Volume 3.* (Casterton: Parthenon Publishing))

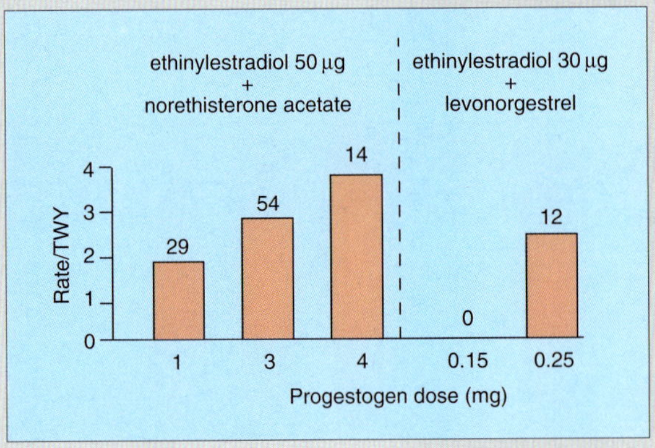

Figure 12.2 Incidence of arterial diseases during oral contraceptive use per 1000 woman-years (TWY). (Adapted from Kay, C. R. (1984). The Royal College of General Practitioners' Oral Contraception Study: some recent observations. *Clin. Obstet. Gynaecol.*, **11**, 759–86)

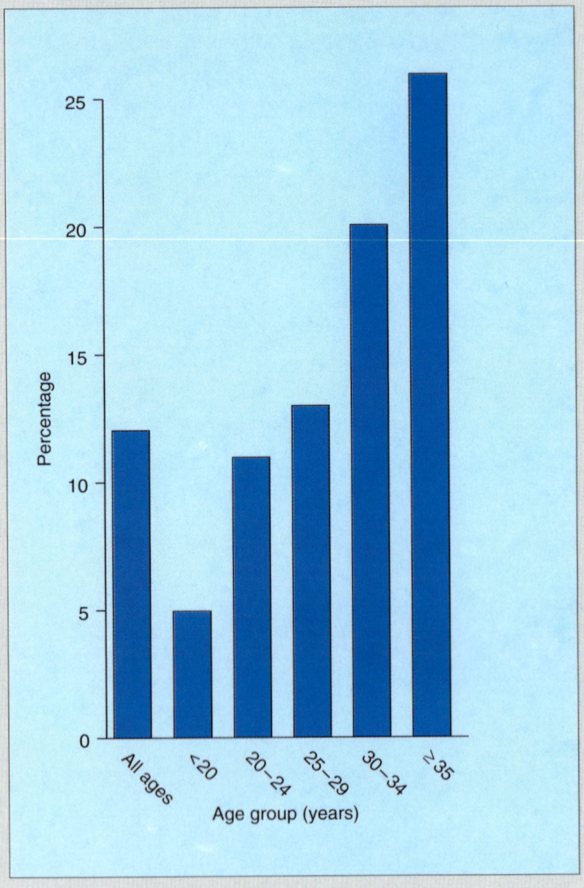

Figure 12.3 Percentage of oral contraceptive users in the USA taking pills with more than 50 μg of estrogen, by age group of women, 1980. (Adapted from Ory, H. W., Forrest, J.D. and Lincoln, R. (1983). *Making Choices: Evaluating Health Risks and Benefits of Birth Control Methods.* (New York: Alan Guttmacher))

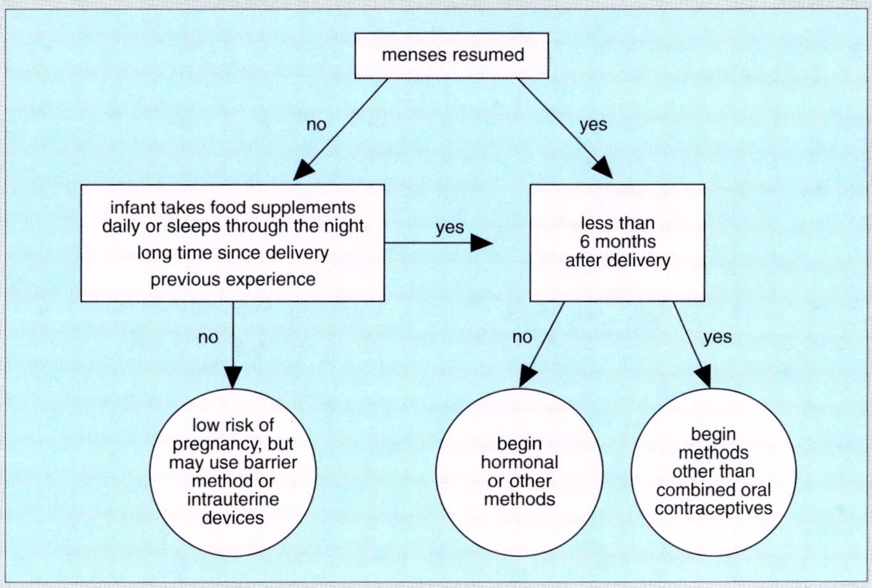

Figure 12.4 A simplified decision tree for the introduction of contraception during breastfeeding. (Adapted from Rosenfield, A. and Fathalla, M. F. (1990). *The Figo Manual of Human Reproduction, Volume 3.* (Casterton: Parthenon Publishing))

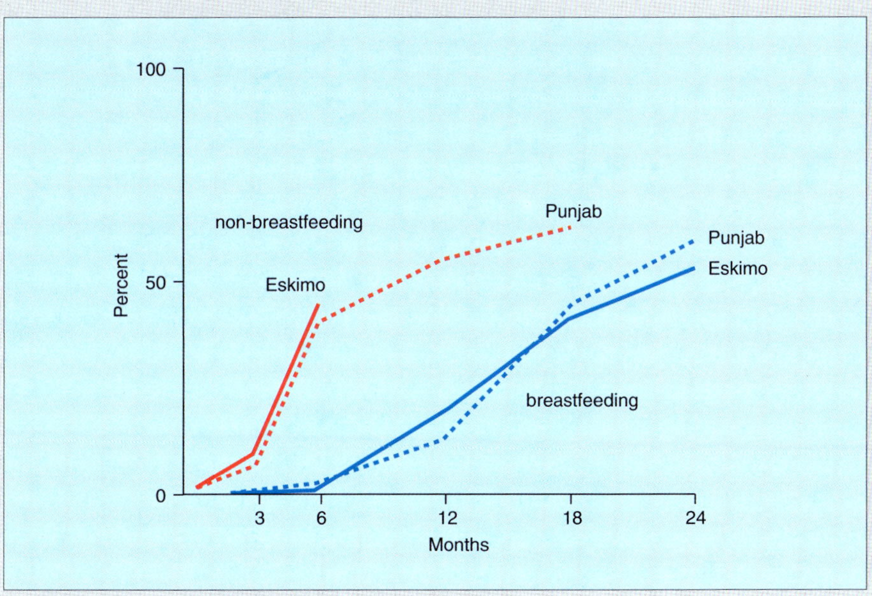

Figure 12.5 Return of menstruation/ovulation in bottle-feeding mothers and breastfeeding mothers

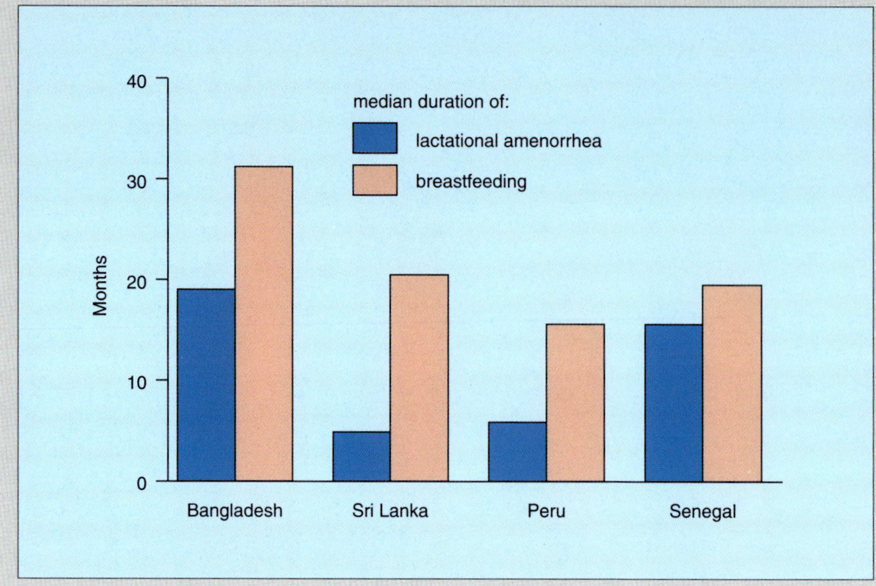

Figure 12.6 Duration of breastfeeding and lactational amenorrhea. (Sources, World Fertility Survey, Bangladesh (1979); Demographic and Health Surveys – Peru (1986), Senegal (1986), Sri Lanka (1987))

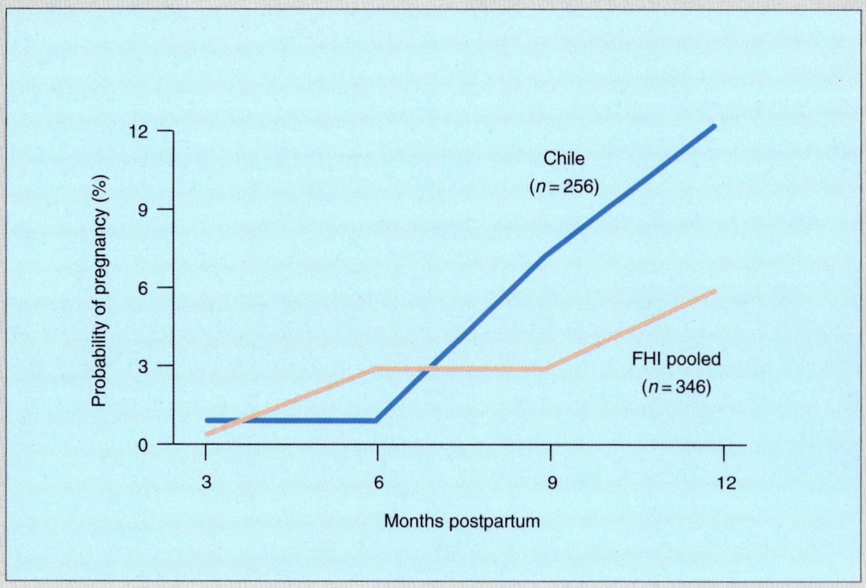

Figure 12.7 Cumulative probability of pregnancy during lactational amenorrhea. (FHI, Family Health International). (Source, Family Health International)

13

Abortion

The term 'abortion' conjures up in one's mind many visions – these include whether it is safe or unsafe, whether it is legal or illegal, whether it causes death or disability, and whether it causes sepsis or hemorrhage. Abortion is controversial and misunderstood.

It is an observed fact that no society has ever achieved a small family size without resorting to abortion – whether legal or illegal. Nevertheless, the number of abortions that occur in a society is highly influenced by access to contraception. Statistics from the Commonwealth of Independent States (previously the USSR), the USA and The Netherlands illustrate this point. All have similar birth rates but in the CIS contraceptives are difficult to obtain and are of poor quality (for good reasons: in the Russian language 'condoms' are 'galoshes'), and voluntary surgical contraception is not offered. As a result, well over 6 million abortions are registered each year. In addition, many doctors take payment from the woman for a slightly less painful and more private operation, and some estimates put the number of abortions in the CIS as high as 12 million/year. In The Netherlands contraceptives are widely available and, although abortion is legal, it is a right that is rarely exercised (Figure 13.1). According to the rate per 1000 fertile women, The Netherlands has one-thirtieth of the abortion rate of the CIS. The USA (which has a slightly smaller population than the CIS) has 1.5 million abortions a year, and lies somewhere between the CIS and The Netherlands in its availability of, and attitudes to, contraception (Figure 13.2).

The majority of the world's population live in countries where abortion is legally available, either on the recommendation of a physician, as in the UK, or at the request of the woman, as in the USA and parts of Eastern Europe.

The problem with abortion is not clinical, but ethical and political. Social surveys show that a minority of people believe abortion is equivalent to murder and should be outlawed. Another minority group believes that women have an unfettered right over their own reproductive systems. Most people are uncomfortable with abortion but recognize that, in many cases, it is the most appropriate solution to the problem. More than 90% of people believe that women ought to be able to have an abortion in cases where the fetus is congenitally abnormal, or the pregnancy follows rape or incest. In 1987, in a secret ballot and by a two to one majority, the people of Ireland voted to amend their Constitution to protect 'the unborn child', yet when in 1992 a 14-year-old girl was pregnant as a result of rape, two-thirds of the population supported her right to travel to London to obtain an abortion. This apparent contradiction is common in many of us and ambivalence towards abortion is hardly surprising. We can, however, learn a great deal from the experience of different countries.

Scientifically, embryologists can no more tell when life begins than an astronomer can tell if heaven exists by looking for the pearly gates with a telescope. The ethical and legal status individuals ascribe to the developing embryo is a matter of belief, not observable fact. In the landmark case Roe vs. Wade 1972, the US Supreme Court wisely stated: 'We need not resolve the difficult question of when life begins. When those trained in the respective disciplines of medicine, philosophy and theology are unable to arrive at a consensus, the judiciary, at this point in the development of man's knowledge, is not in a position to speculate as to the answer.' In other words, abortion is a topic of belief, and therefore of religious tolerance. Society must accommodate a variety of beliefs about life before birth, just as it does about life after death: it should be no more surprising to find an abortion clinic in a city where a significant number of people believe abortion to be murder than it is to find a mosque, a synagogue and a church – all of which teach different pathways to eternal life – in the same community.

As has been shown, the principal defence against abortion is access to good contraception. Laws prohibiting abortion do not seem to make an impact on the numbers of abortions taking place, but raise the danger to the individual woman immeasurably, as well as creating opportunities for financial and sexual exploitation.

Indeed, whilst those who oppose abortion normally do so for well-intentioned humanitarian and ethical considerations, in terms of human suffering and increased mortality, strict anti-abortion laws can lead to very counter-productive results – especially when harshly applied by unresponsive regimes. For example, Nicolae Ceausescu introduced strict abortion law in Romania in 1966; 9 months later the birth rate doubled, but with the passage of time a criminal abortion network was established in the country and the birth rate fell back to previous levels, although the maternal mortality rate rose to the highest in Europe (Figure 13.3). Thousands – perhaps tens of thousands of women died from botched abortions during Ceausescu's regime. In the year following the death of Ceausescu and the liberalization of abortion, maternal mortality fell by 55% as unsafe abortions began to disappear.

In contrast, in 1993 Poland reversed its previously liberal abortion laws, and experience suggests that as a result, deaths may be expected to rise in the 1990s.

In the nineteenth century, the Scottish obstetrician James Young Simpson described a vacuum technique which he appears to have used to induce early abortions. Working independently and outside the medical profession, Harvey Karman, a California psychologist, developed a flexible plastic cannula with hand-held syringe (Figure 13.4). This is now widely used in many countries and is a safe, simple way of performing early abortion, whether done under paracervical block or even without any anesthetic at all. Vacuum aspiration is now considered the optimal way of inducing abortion in the first trimester of pregnancy.

Technically, early abortion is a simple, safe procedure which, when done with modern techniques, is four or five times as safe as carrying a pregnancy to term. All abortions have greater side-effects and risks of death the longer the duration of the pregnancy. Abortion in the first 12 weeks of pregnancy is considered safer than carrying the pregnancy to term. By about the 22nd week of pregnancy, the risks of performing an abortion exceed those of carrying a pregnancy to term (Figure 13.5).

In the first 8 weeks of pregnancy, the uterus can be emptied using a small flexible plastic cannula a little bigger than a drinking straw. Local anesthesia is usually appropriate. After 12 weeks of pregnancy, the operation is clinically more difficult and ethically more challenging. Even so, the long-term follow-up of women who have had abortions has not demonstrated any consistent adverse psychological or physical effects.

One woman a minute dies in the world from pregnancy, childbirth or abortion. The mortality rate per 100 000 legal abortions, for selected countries during selected periods of time is illustrated in

Figure 13.6. Badly performed abortions are up to 1000 times more dangerous than early vacuum aspiration abortion.

Figure 13.7 shows how the problems associated with abortion have decreased as the use of contraceptives has increased.

The dangers of abortion are hemorrhage, infection and perforation of the uterus. In parts of Latin America, botched abortion places the largest single demand on the blood transfusion services. In most months in one hospital in Addis Ababa, Ethiopia, more women die from the consequences of illegal abortion than die in the whole of Great Britain from legal abortion in one year.

Techniques of unsafe abortion include pushing foreign bodies through the neck of the womb, taking dangerous poisons such as ergot or quinine, and physical trauma to the abdomen until the placenta and fetus are dislodged (Figure 13.8). Physical violence is cited as a cause of abortion in the Bible (*Exodus* 21: 22) where, incidentally, it is considered a crime but not murder.

All societies have a variety of abortion techniques, from the use of drugs to the insertion of foreign bodies into the cervix. In Latin America a urinary catheter, or 'sonda', pushed through the cervix is a common method of mechanical abortion. Umbrella ribs, the proverbial coat hanger (Figure 13.9) and sticks, twigs, roots and even condoms that are inserted into the uterus and then filled with water have all been used to terminate pregnancy in some countries of the developing world where abortion is illegal. In Brazil, women have used a prostaglandin (Cytotec®), available in pharmacies to treat gastric ulcers to initiate uterine bleeding, and then relied on the hospital to complete the 'inevitable abortion'.

RU 486 (mifepristone) is an antiprogestational drug which was first used in France in the 1980s. When administered with prostaglandin it will induce an abortion in the first 6 weeks of pregnancy. RU 486 also appears to work well as an emergency contraceptive although this use is not generally approved in any country. RU 486 is the first medically effective method of abortion to gain approval; however, its use is controversial and carefully controlled.

The issue of abortion generated a great deal of acrimonious debate at the Cairo International Conference on Population and Development held from 5–13 September, 1994. The Draft Program of Action in its Chapter 8 addressed the issue of unsafe abortion as a public health problem. The particular paragraph which had the most amount of discussion with regard to abortion was paragraph 8.25. The modified and accepted version is shown below:

'In no case should abortion be promoted as a method of family planning. All Governments and relevant intergovernmental and non-governmental organizations are urged to strengthen their commitment to women's health, to deal with the health impact of unsafe abortion as a major public health concern and to reduce the recourse to abortion through expanded and improved family planning services. Prevention of unwanted pregnancies must always be given the highest priority and all attempts should be made to eliminate the need for abortion. Women who have unwanted pregnancies should have ready access to reliable information and compassionate counseling. Any measures or changes related to abortion within the health system can only be determined at the national or local level according to the national legislative process. In circumstances in which abortion is not against the law, such abortion should be safe. In all cases, women should have access to quality services for the management of complications arising from abortion. Post-abortion counseling, education and family planning services should be offered promptly which will also help to avoid repeat abortions.' The footnote reads: 'Unsafe abortion is defined as a procedure for terminating an unwanted pregnancy either by persons lacking necessary skills or in an environment lacking the minimal medical standards or both.'

Africa

Algeria
Angola
Benin
Botswana
Burkina Faso
Burundi
Cameroon
Cent. Af. Rep.
Chad
Congo
Côte d'Ivoire
Egypt
Ethiopia
Gabon
Ghana
Guinea
Kenya
Lesotho
Liberia
Libya
Madagascar
Malawi
Mali
Mauritania
Mauritius
Morocco
Mozambique
Namibia
Niger
Nigeria
Rwanda
Senegal
Sierra Leone
Somalia
South Africa
Sudan
Tanzania
Togo
Tunisia
Uganda
Zaire
Zambia
Zimbabwe

Asia & Oceania

Afghanistan
Australia
Bangladesh
Cambodia
China
Hong Kong
India
Indonesia
Iran
Iraq
Israel
Japan
Jordan
Korea, Dem. Rep.
Korea, Rep. of
Kuwait
Laos
Lebanon
Malaysia
Mongolia
Myanmat (Burma)
Nepal
New Zealand
Oman
Pakistan
Papua New Guinea
Philippines
Saudi Arabia
Singapore
Sri Lanka
Syria
Taiwan
Thailand
Turkey
UAE
Vietnam
Yemen

The Americas

Argentina
Bolivia
Brazil
Canada
Chile
Colombia
Costa Rica
Cuba
Dominican Rep.
Ecuador
El Salvador
Guatemala
Guyana
Haiti
Honduras
Jamaica
Mexico
Nicaragua
Panama
Paraguay
Peru
Puerto Rico
Trinidad & Tob.
United States
Uruguay
Venezuela

Europe

Albania
Austria
Belgium
Bulgaria
Czech. Rep.
Denmark
Finland
France
Germany
Great Britain
Greece
Hungary
Iceland
Ireland
Italy
The Netherlands
Norway
Northern Ireland
Poland
Portugal
Romania
USSR (former)
Spain
Sweden
Switzerland
Yugoslavia (former)

There are four types of abortion laws

Very strict – to save a woman's life or under no circumstances

Rather strict – maternal health and/or judicial reasons (rape, incest)

Rather broad – social and social-medical reasons

On request – reasons not specified or on request

Figure 13.1 Abortion laws worldwide. Note, the above classification is intended as a general indicator only, and is not intended to be a precise summary of the legal situation in each country – since details of the law currently in force will differ significantly within the same broad classification band

Annual number	36–53 million
Rate per 1000 women, aged 15–44 years	32–46
Lifetime abortion incidence per woman	0.9–1.3
Abortions as % of conceptions	21–28%
Lowest known rate *(The Netherlands)*	5 per 1000 women
Highest known rate *(Romania, 1990)*	188 per 1000 women

Figure 13.2 Worldwide incidence of induced abortion

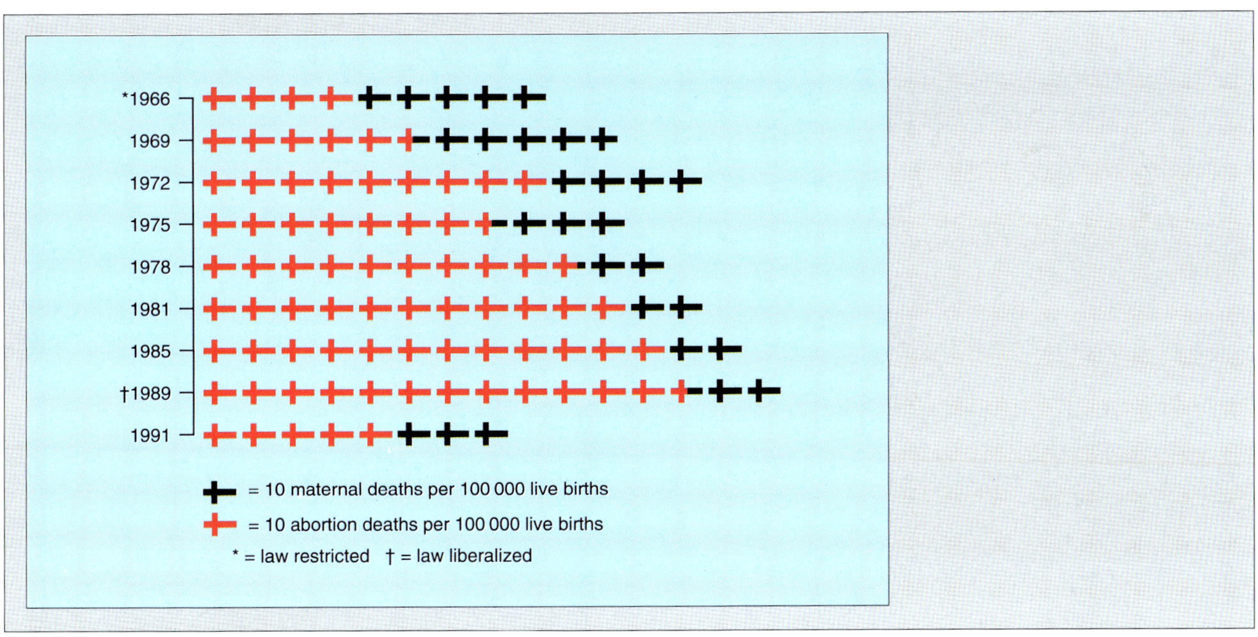

Figure 13.3 Abortion rates and maternal mortality (Romania 1960–1990)

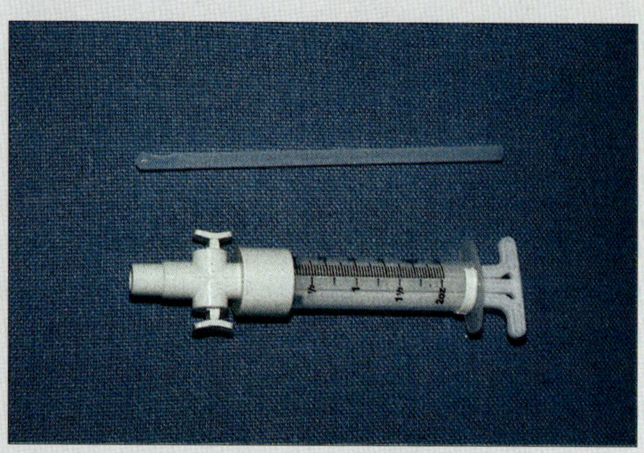

Figure 13.4 Hand-held vacuum syringe and Karman cannula. (Source, International Projects Assistance Services, USA)

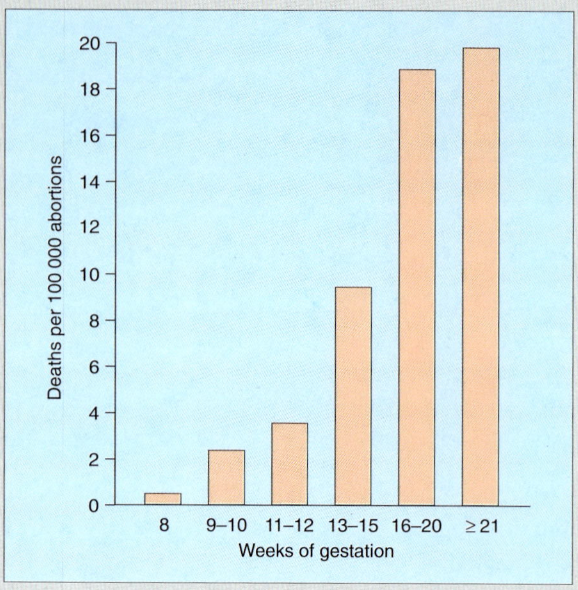

Figure 13.5 Mortality related to legal abortion, by week of gestation, compared with the risk of carrying a pregnancy to term (note that maternal mortality could be as high as 5–600/100 000 live births in some developing countries)

Country	*Mortality rate*	*% decrease*
Canada *(1970/75–1976/83)*	3.6 – 0.2	94.0%
Czechoslovakia (*1957/66–1976/83)*	3.8 – 0.4	89.0%
Denmark *(1940/50–1976/87*	195 – 0.7	99.6%
England/Wales *(1968/69–1980/87)*	26 – 1.3	95.0%
Hungary *(1957/62–1968/78)*	4.1 – 0.7	83.0%
Sweden *(1946/48–1980/87)*	250 – 0.4	99.8%
USA *(1970–1980/85)*	19 – 0.6	97.0%

Figure 13.6 Mortality rate per 100 000 legal abortions, for selected countries during selected periods of time

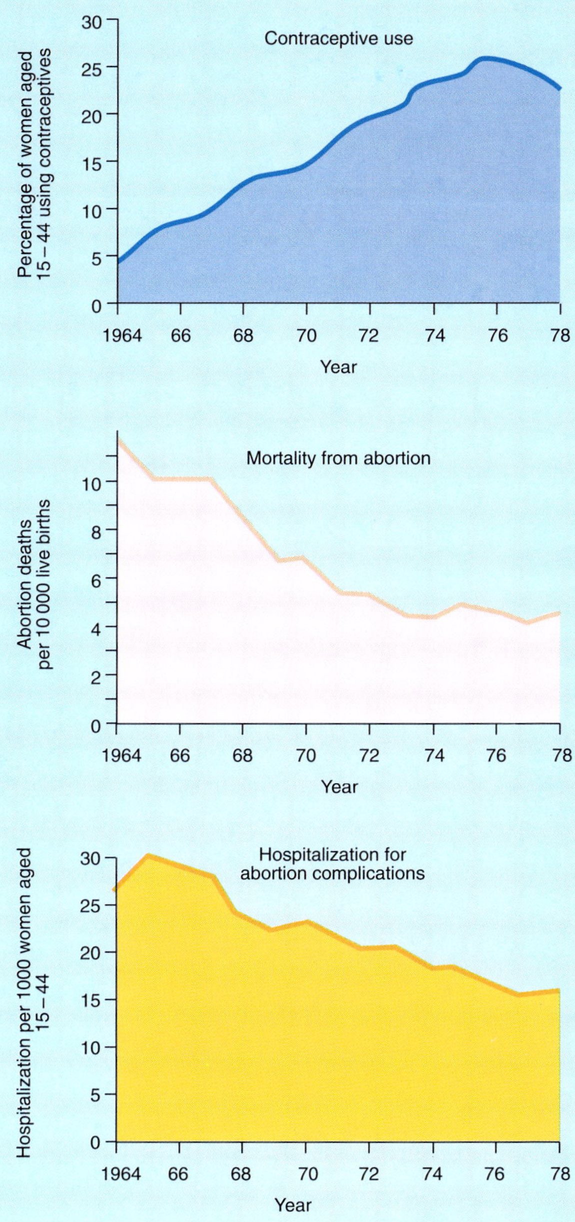

Figure 13.7 Problems from abortion decline as use of contraceptives increases, Chile 1964-78. (Source, *Preventing Maternal Death.* (1989). (World Health Organization))

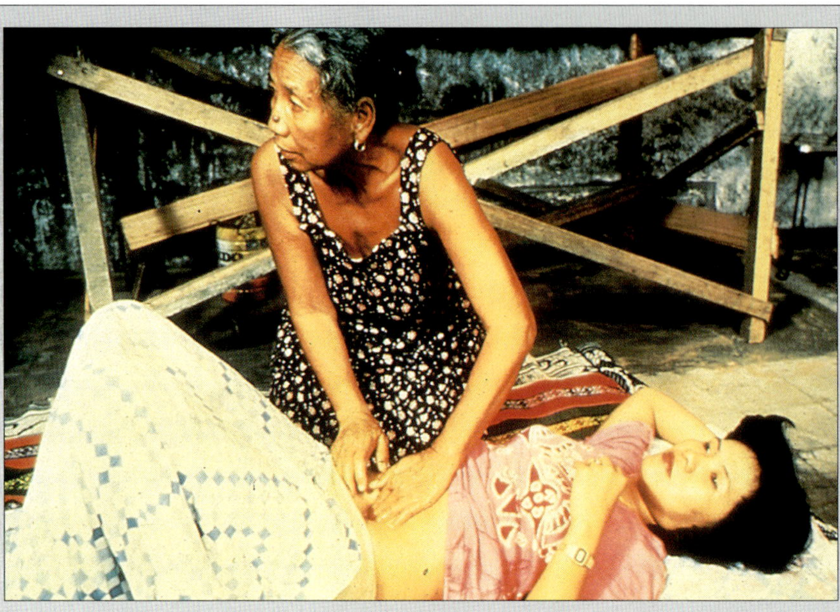

Figure 13.8 An illegal abortion demonstration in the Philippines

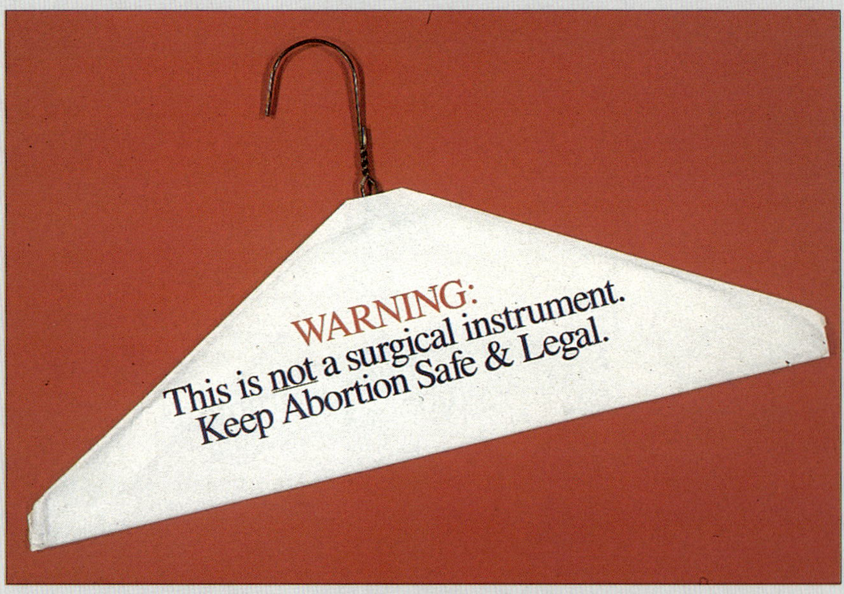

Figure 13.9 A coat hanger, which, in some countries of the developing world where abortion is illegal, is inserted into the uterus to terminate pregnancy

14

AIDS

Acquired immune deficiency syndrome (AIDS) was first described as a clinical entity at the beginning of the 1980s. Figure 14.1 illustrates the sequence of the formation of a human immunodeficiency virus (HIV) particle, the causative agent of AIDS, at the surface of an infected lymphocyte. It is incurable and apparently universally lethal. A great deal of research has been carried out in the search for a suitable vaccine, but none is immediately in sight.

AIDS is changing the face of family planning. AIDS prevention uses condoms and, more importantly, the same range of political and counseling skills that has been used in the development of family planning services. The virus is fragile and relatively difficult to transmit from one human being to another. The good news about HIV is that it is not transmitted by coughing and sneezing like its cousin the common cold retrovirus, but only in semen and blood. Modes of transmission of HIV include blood transfusion, intravenous drug use, mother to fetus transmission, and anal, vaginal and oral intercourse. The most common mode of transmission is sexual.

Figure 14.2 shows the global importance of each major route of HIV infection. Sexual transmission was responsible for 86% of HIV infection, with a homosexual : heterosexual ratio of 5:1 (anal intercourse is more likely to transmit the virus than vaginal and vaginal more likely than oral). The presence of certain sexually transmissible diseases substantially encourages the spread at intercourse. It is possible but not certain that circumcised men are less likely to acquire the disease than uncircumcised men.

Blood-borne transmission, particularly from needle sharing by intravenous drug users, is an exceptionally high-risk activity and sometimes, drug users represent one of the first core groups to become infected as the disease spreads (as occurred in Thailand in the late 1980s).

Diseases, like people, have a reproductive rate (Figure 14.3) – that is, how many people a person with the disease will infect before they die or recover. If the reproductive rate is above one, the disease spreads; if it is below one it will fade out. In Africa and parts of Asia the reproductive rate for HIV infection is above one and spread is rapid. Among many heterosexual communities in the West it may be below one, which means that clusters of infection will occur by spread from groups with high-risk behaviors (e.g. intravenous drug users) although a self-sustaining epidemic is less likely. This means that even relatively small changes in behavior, condom use or sexually transmissible disease control could have a marked effect on the overall epidemic (Figure 14.4).

There are three things that can be done to slow the spread of HIV:

(1) Educate about the nature of the disease and the need to avoid multiple sex partners;

(2) Ensure easy availability of condoms; and

(3) Treat other sexually transmissible diseases.

Studies have shown that most people have relatively few sexual partners in a lifetime (Figure 14.5); a few have large numbers.

These three interventions act synergistically. There is a tremendous advantage in creating interventions as early as possible in the history of the epidemic (Figure 14.6) and focusing on those individuals at highest risk of acquiring and transmitting the disease, namely prostitutes and homosexual men. AIDS has created a great deal of fear and discrimination against people with the virus. It has also produced inspiring examples of leadership, compassion, community support and peer education.

HIV infection never killed anyone. Death occurs as a result of opportunistic infections which occur as natural immunity crumbles as the result of HIV infection which selectively attacks T cells in the lymphoid system.

AIDS is a global pandemic and by the year 2000 more people will be infected with the virus than were killed as combatants and civilians in the Second World War. Despite this tragic loss of life, AIDS will have little impact on population growth. The 40 million people likely to die from AIDS in the first decade of the 21st century will be equivalent to less than 6 months' population growth in that same 10 years.

Globally, too little money is being spent on preventing the spread of AIDS. The estimated global cost of AIDS prevention and care for 1990 was $3.9 billion. Of this amount, affluent countries account for 93% of the total cost; care in affluent countries accounts for 60% of total costs (Figure 14.7).

Latex condoms significantly interrupt vaginal and anal transmission, but small numbers of virus particles the size of HIV have been shown to traverse the membrane of many commercially available condoms, although the clinical significance of such leakage is uncertain. Perhaps the greatest immediate need is for a vaginal spermicide/virucide which a woman could use when she suspects a partner may have risked acquiring HIV but she cannot compel him to use a condom. Several candidate chemicals already exist (nonoxynol-9, chlorhexidine, benzylchonium chloride and even dextran) but the formulation of an acceptable preparation would be critical. It would be essential to demonstrate that any preparation does not damage the vaginal epithelium or cervix, because if it did it might accelerate rather than retard transmission.

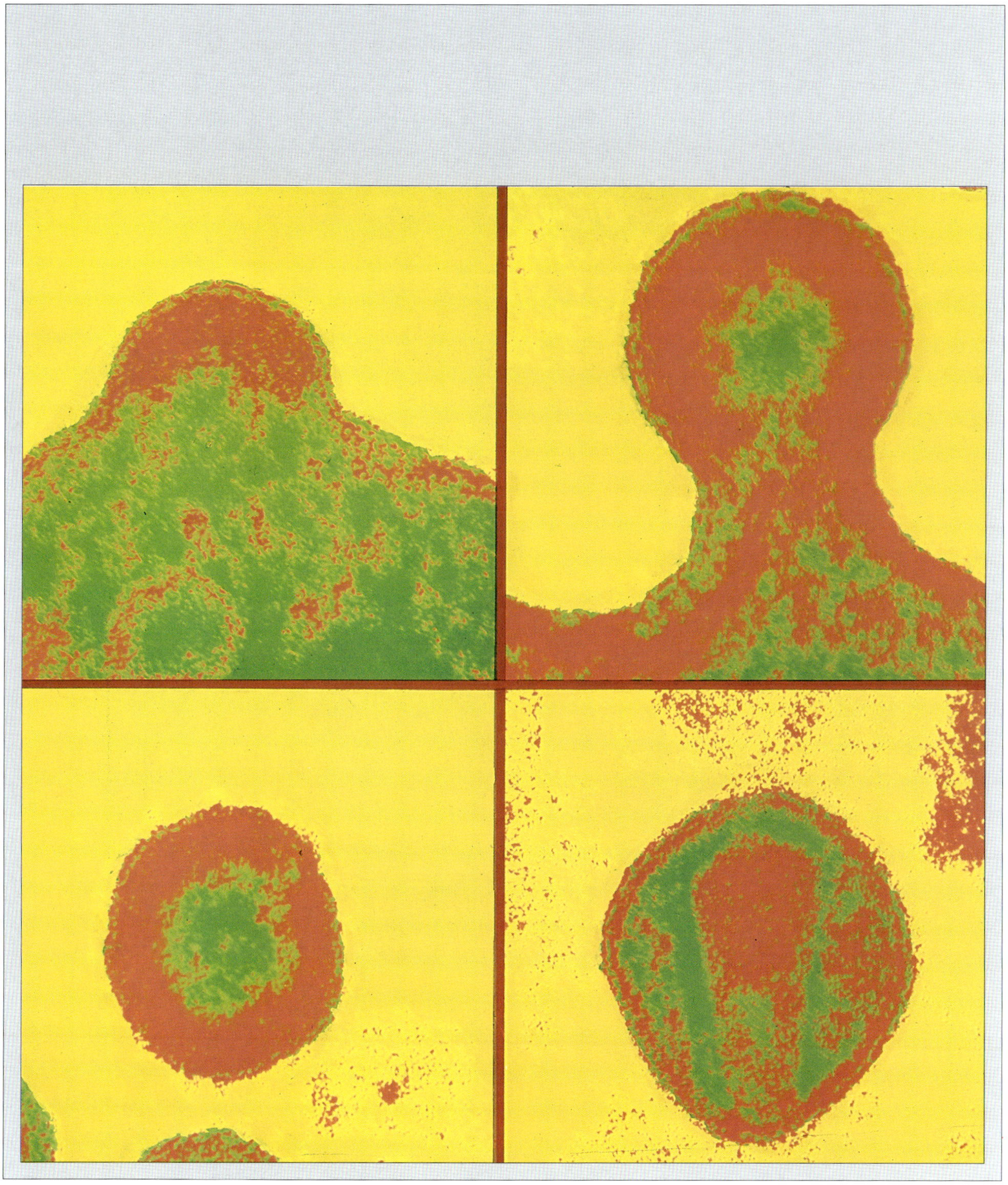

Figure 14.1 Formation of an AIDS virus particle. The sequence shows the formation of the HIV particle, the causative agent of AIDS on the surface of an infected lymphocyte. (Source, Science Photo Library, London, UK)

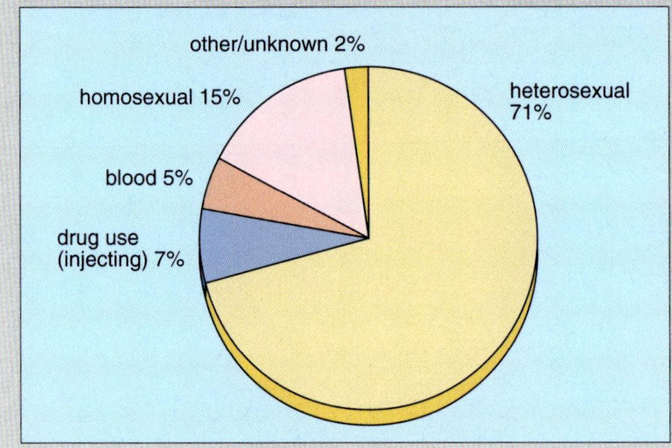

Figure 14.2 Proportion of cumulative adult HIV infections and mode of transmission

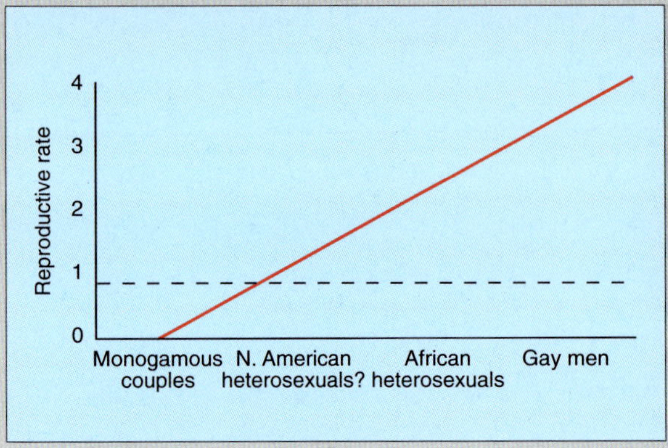

Figure 14.3 Reproductive rate of HIV

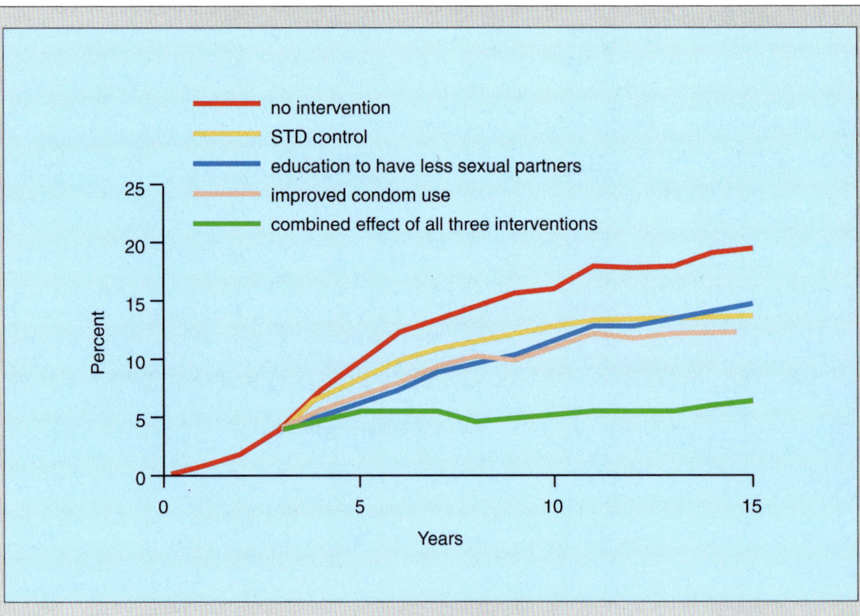

Figure 14.4 Computer model of the impact of education, condom use and treatment of sexually transmissible diseases on the spread of AIDS; individually, each intervention has little impact but all three together have a powerful effect. (STD, sexually transmissible disease)

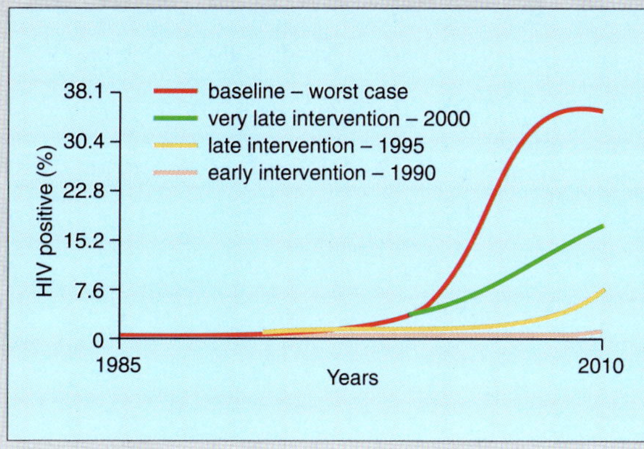

Figure 14.6 Computer model of the impact of interventions by the time the interventions are started after the beginning of an epidemic in a country. (Source, Family Health International)

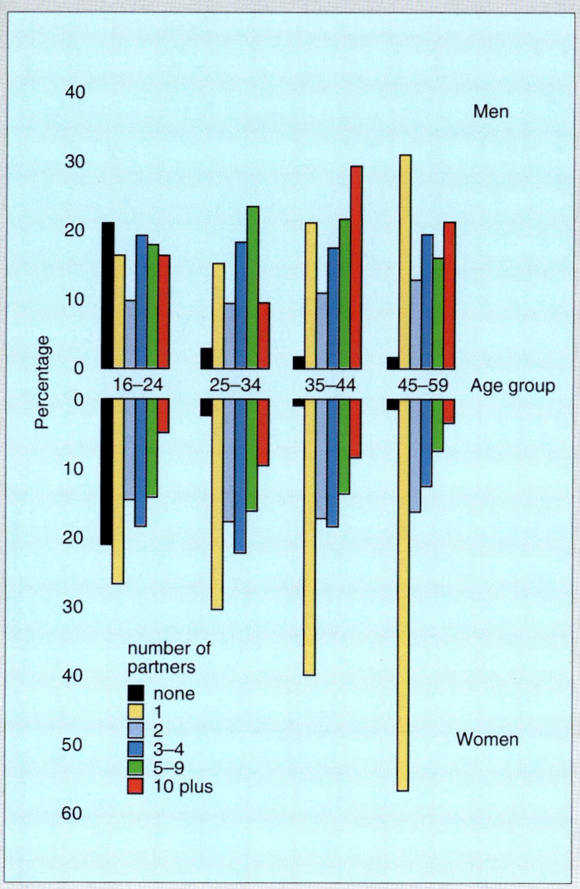

Figure 14.5 AIDS spreads partly because human sexual behavior is heterogeneous. (Data from the UK Survey of Sexual Behaviour, 1992)

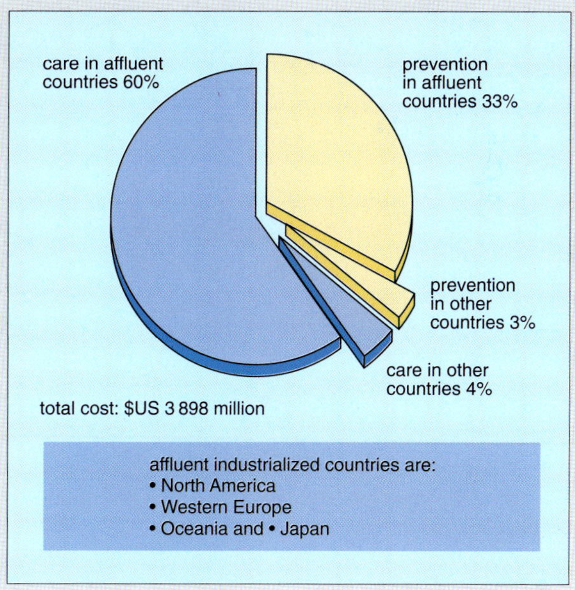

Figure 14.7 Estimated global costs of AIDS prevention and care in the world, 1990. Share by affluent and other countries

15

New methods on the horizon

CONTRACEPTIVE DEVELOPMENT

Contraceptive development is a long, slow, expensive, uncertain process (Figure 15.1). Thousands of chemical entities need to be screened before any are found effective, even in experimental animals. Of those methods which pass laboratory testing, very few are safe enough to be tested on human volunteers. In phase I clinical trials, a few tens of individuals in carefully controlled situations are given the candidate drug or device for short-term use. In phase II clinical trials a few hundred volunteers may use the method, primarily to discover any short-term hazards. In phase III clinical trials of a contraceptive, an aggregate of at least 600 woman-years of exposure is achieved and the goal is to measure effectiveness and gather additional information on short-term side-effects. Once a drug has been approved for marketing it is essential to continue postmarketing surveillance (sometimes called phase IV clinical trials). If, for example, the drug has a serious adverse effect in one in 10 000 or one in 100 000, then it may require several million woman-years of exposure before the risk is observed and measured. In today's world, it may cost 200 million dollars or more to bring a drug from a laboratory to the market-place (Figure 15.2). The US National Academy of Science has recently suggested that the requirements for premarketing testing of drugs might be somewhat simplified and a greater investment, including perhaps a contribution from the pharmaceutical industry, should be made in postmarketing surveillance. Postmarketing surveillance takes several years to implement, so when drugs or devices are improved (as has happened with pills and IUDs), there is often a long interval when today's methods continue to be assessed on yesterday's statistics.

Species differences in reproduction are much wider than, say, for the cardiovascular system. Giving a contraceptive in several times the human dose to primates for long intervals is part of drug development but it remains an imperfect model of human physiology. In the last analysis, all new drugs and devices constitute an experiment on our own species. A great deal of patient and prudent work can be done to make the introduction of a new drug as safe as possible but there is no way to eliminate all unforeseen risks. All manipulation of the reproductive system in the prevention of unwanted pregnancy involves possible hazards and these are being reflected by exceedingly high malpractice insurance rates in the USA in recent years – one reason why contraceptive pills in the USA cost 10–12 dollars a cycle while the same products can be bought internationally in bulk for about 20 cents.

In the past there have been some companies within the pharmaceutical industry which were active in real innovative research and development. Today, it is mainly two companies working in this field, namely Organon and Schering.

IMPROVING EXISTING METHODS

Over recent decades, improvements in existing methods have often been more important than the introduction of new methods. For example, today's IUDs and oral contraceptives are so different from the first generation of these methods introduced in the 1960s that they almost count as new methods. Incremental improvements in design are most likely when comparative studies of different methods are conducted by independent observers, as has happened with IUDs. When first introduced, the pill used almost as much hormone in each tablet as today's user receives in a month and, as a consequence of this reduction, cardiovascular risks have been greatly reduced or even eliminated. Copper- and progestin-releasing IUDs have lower pregnancy rates and fewer side-effects than the inert plastic devices introduced 30 years ago, and the progestin-containing IUDs may actually reduce, rather than increase the risk of pelvic inflammatory disease. The new levonorgestrel IUD also has a protective effect against the occurrence of ectopic pregnancy. New copper-bearing IUDs, for example, Flexigard 330® (Figure 15.3) may reduce the incidence of side-effects.

Oral contraceptive doses are unlikely to be lowered further, although new synthetic hormones may be synthesized. New implants and injectables are possible: subdermal implants with one rod instead of six would be a step forward and a biodegradable implant, that did not require removal, would be welcome. Steroid hormones are rapidly absorbed through the vaginal wall and even the ordinary pill has been used this way. This method of delivery bypasses the liver and has some advantages over oral use, reducing, for example, complaints of nausea. Silastic vaginal rings containing hormones have been used as successful contraceptives in WHO sponsored trials. The levonorgestrel IUD, the subdermal implant – NORPLANT-2 and a contraceptive ring are illustrated in Figure 15.4. Unfortunately, even simple improvements are sometimes too costly to introduce past modern drug regulatory authorities: for example, the addition of small quantities of testosterone to an injectable progestin would correct the risk of osteoporosis and reduced libido associated with the method.

New IUDs, such as the device by Wildermersch in Belgium, which anchors a thread with copper sleeves in the uterus but does away with a rigid framework may represent an important advance. Even new condoms, such as loose-fitting plastic devices, could improve the range of contraceptive choices.

DEVELOPING NEW METHODS

In the 1960s, when condoms and coitus interruptus were the most common methods, family planning leaders were pleading for research on female methods. Today, the cry is often to introduce a 'male pill'. WHO trials of a male systemic method using testosterone have been conducted. Testosterone is made in the Leydig cells in the testis and sperm production is only possible in an environment exposed to high levels of testosterone. If testosterone is given by injection then the pituitary gonadotropins are inhibited and, while the levels of circulating testosterone are adequate for all the other aspects of male behavior, levels in the testis fall so low that sperm production stops. It takes 120 days to make a sperm, so male systemic methods take some time to act and some time to reverse. In the case of women, systemically active methods imitate the natural process of ovulation inhibition occurring with pregnancy and lactation, but in the case of the man there is no natural interruption of fertility to imitate. Therefore, there are no biological reasons for assuming a male systemic method might have any advantages of the sort associated with the pill and reduction of cancer. High doses of testosterone, however, can cause aggressive behavior in men. A variety of chemicals have been tried that prevent sperm production or interfere with specific components of sperm activity, such as acrosome function, but none have reached phase II or III human trials.

Hypothalamic releasing hormones have been well studied in women and men and are relatively easy to synthesize. At first glance, they offer little advantage over pituitary hormones, other than interrupting the same reproductive processes at a different location. However, Pike and his co-workers in Los Angeles are conducting phase II trials of a combination of hypothalamic releasing and ovarian hormones, designed not only to inhibit fertility but to change the hormonal environment of the breast in such a way as to reduce the risk of cancer later in life. In The Netherlands, Cohen is approaching the same issue by combining the pineal hormone melatonin with ovarian steroids, based on the observation that women with breast cancer often have lower melatonin levels than healthy women. It will require time and large-scale use to demonstrate if either of these approaches reduces breast cancer, but if either succeeds, it is likely to form the basis of a new generation of fundamentally different and profoundly important therapies for the twenty-first century.

Some thought has been given to the possible immunological control of fertility. Unlike antibodies against infective organisms, an immunological method of contraception must be active against a protein essential to fertility but not having any other natural function. Two components have been investigated in animals. The first are the gonadotropic hormones formed in the placenta during pregnancy, which are essential to reproduction, but which differ immunologically from the gonadotropins manufactured in the pituitary, and some small-scale human trials have been conducted by Talwar in India and other researchers. The zona pellucida, which surrounds the egg, is a unique structure, and Atkin in Scotland, for example, has successfully interrupted fertility in primates by immunizing with anti-zona vaccines.

Unfortunately, the monies going into new methods such as vaccines are insufficient to bring about any real revolution in family planning in the near future. Probably the best that can be hoped for is a slow but steady improvement in current methods and perhaps some new barrier methods to fill the need mentioned earlier for a method women could use to protect themselves against HIV and other sexually transmissible disease transmissions.

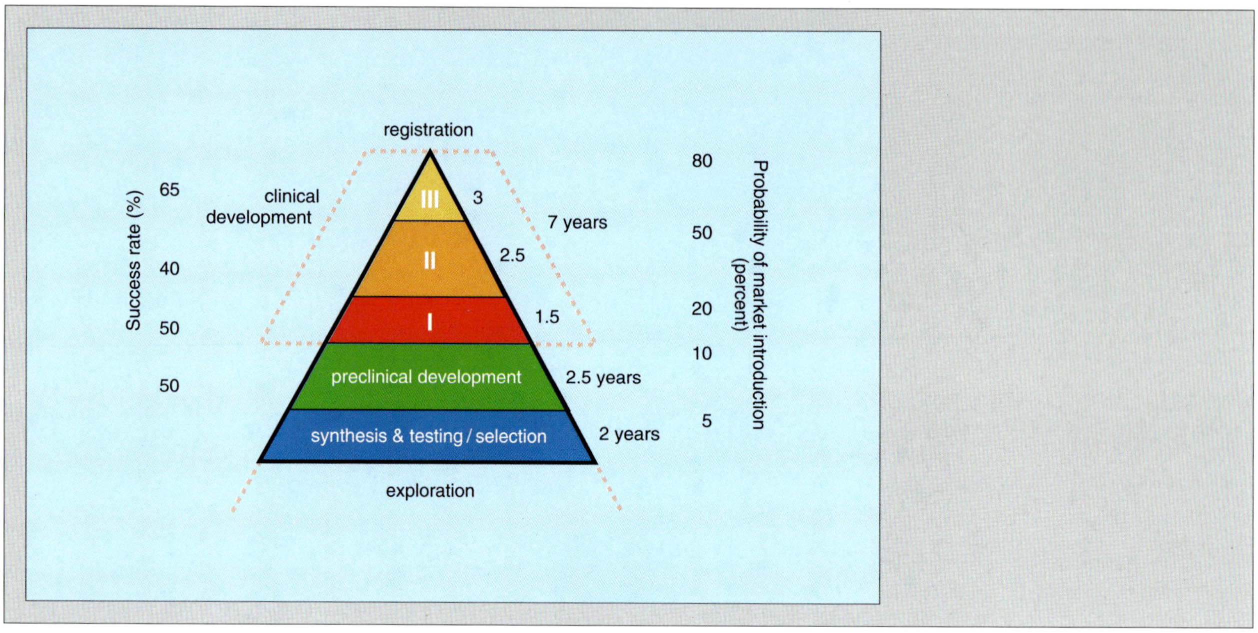

Figure 15.1 Time and risks involved in pharmaceutical research and development. (Courtesy of Professor H. Vemer, N. V. Organon, Oss, The Netherlands)

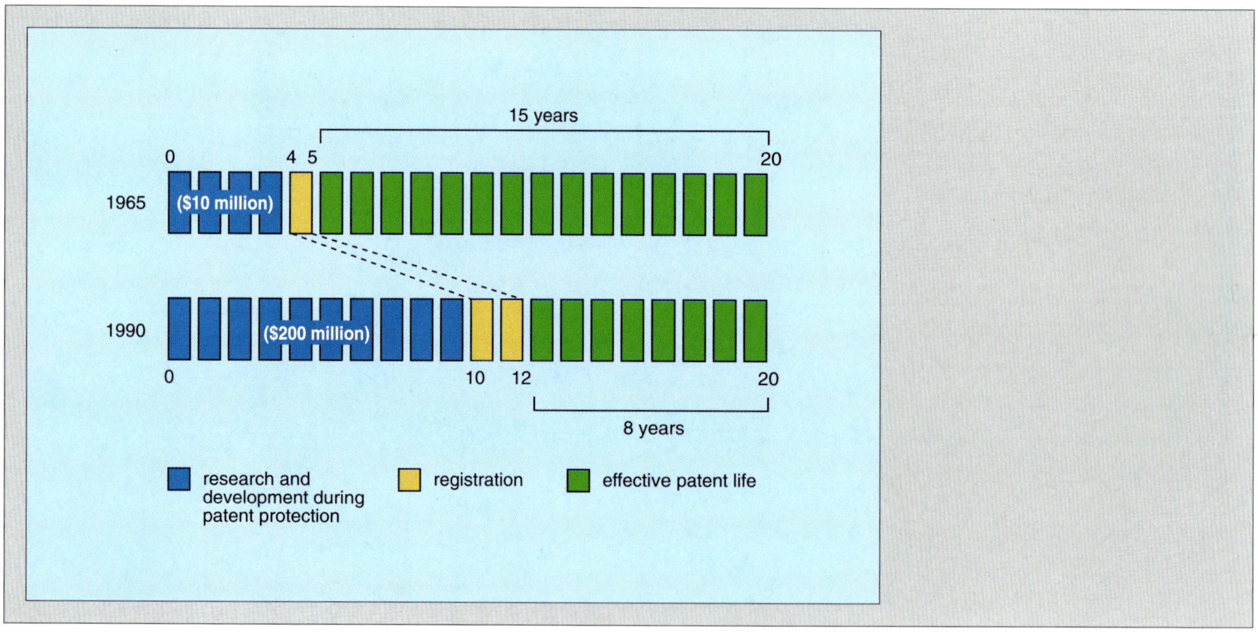

Figure 15.2 Effective patent life of medicines (1965–1990). (Courtesy of Professor H. Vemer, N. V. Organon, Oss, The Netherlands)

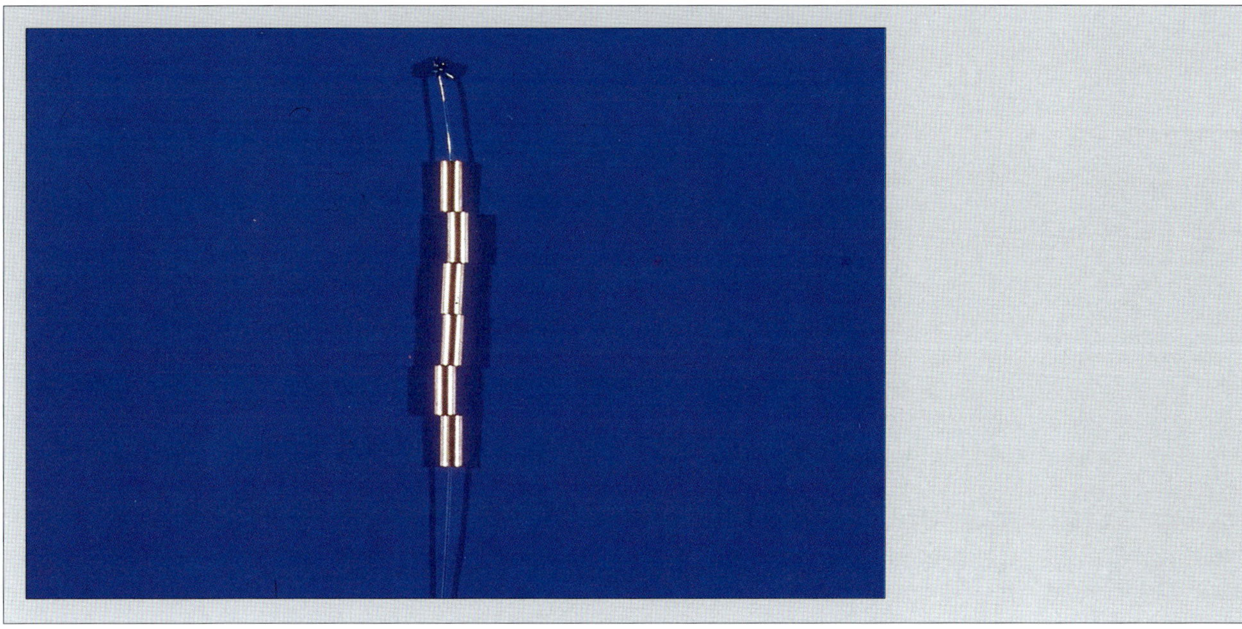

Figure 15.3 Flexigard 330®, a new copper-bearing IUD

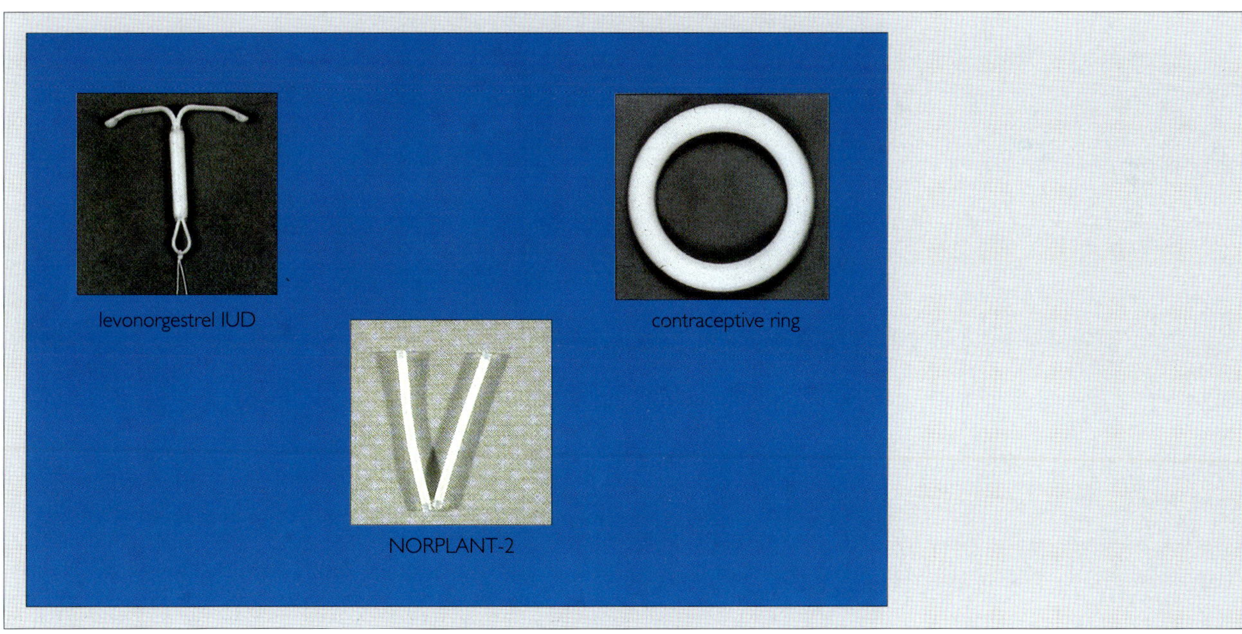

Figure 15.4 Examples of contraceptive methods recently developed. (Source, Population Council, New York, USA)

16

Conclusions

Those who believe reproductive freedom is a basic human right are beginning to emerge from a long dark tunnel: for the first time in human history, there are one or two areas of the world where women enjoy social equality with men, sexual autonomy and freedom of reproductive choice. In other, larger areas of the world change is occurring and progress is being made, but elsewhere hundreds of millions of women remain disadvantaged, often exploited and sometimes emotionally or physically abused. Where women are unjustly treated, men cannot reach their full potential either.

It may take generations before the bonds of tradition are broken in some places. Fortunately, family planning choices can be made available relatively quickly and in almost any culture, from the Islamic areas of South Asia, where many women are in purdah, to the single mother with a series of partners, encountered in the Caribbean. While access to family planning cannot solve social or economic problems, it can lighten the heavy burdens laid on people – especially women – by their circumstances. Indeed, surveys have shown that millions of women do not want more children (Figure 16.1). Reductions in the rate of childbearing have been especially rapid in East and South-east Asia, as well as in Latin America (Figure 16.2). The pace and extent to which family planning choices are expanded will not only have a profound impact on the reproductive health of these individuals, but also have an important relationship with other global problems, particularly related to the environment and to the huge task of moving the global economy from its present dependence on fossil fuels to one that is biologically sustainable.

The difficulty of recreating the cloying conservatism that held back family planning in the Western world until the second half of the twentieth century has been emphasized earlier. In the 1920s, Aldous Huxley said of his contemporary world, 'In most countries, the only state-supported orthodoxy is sexual orthodoxy'. Only the strongest and most charismatic of personalities were able to break through the formidable barriers which society had built between individuals and their reproductive freedoms. Those who fought for family planning were not always likeable people: Marie Stopes was a prima donna who frequently quarreled with her colleagues, Helena Wright had an eccentric belief in spiritualism, and Margaret Sanger, like all of us, was a prisoner of her own time when it came to writing about eugenics and 'illiterates, paupers, unemployables, criminals, prostitutes, dope-fiends' whom she felt should be separated from the rest of society to 'improve their moral conduct' and prevent them reproducing.

As late as 1952, at the time of the foundation of the International Planned Parenthood Federation, a distinguished scientist, Professor Joseph Needham, believed only compulsion would lower fertility in some countries. It was so difficult and so unusual to talk openly about family planning that more than one generation of demographers and sociologists grew up ignoring contraception and abortion, as variables in fertility!

Differentials in fertility between different social groups or different countries were explained by differences in education, income and other correlates which were studied so intensively. It followed that, if these differentials could not be removed, there would have to be some degree of coercion. The glorious discovery of the past quarter century has been that, when individuals of any social, ethnic, or cultural background are given genuine choices, then the overwhelming majority do not choose to have more children than their love and physical resources can support. The 'unemployables', whose large families worried Margaret Sanger, were simply those who had even less opportunity than their neighbors of jumping over the many hurdles separating them from the family planning services that they needed. The rapid growth of developing countries that worried Joseph Needham was, to a considerable extent, a manifestation of the fact that the Europeans denied their colonies access to family planning, even more thoroughly than they tried to deny it to their own citizens.

The light at the end of the tunnel is growing brighter but is still some way off. Contemporary family planning policies are often muddled. Some decision-makers still repeat yesterday's mistakes and assume that fertility will not decline until other variables, such as education and income, are improved. Obviously, family planning moves more rapidly in a world where people are literate and prosperous, but socio-economic progress is not a prerequisite of a falling birth rate. Even in the West, research shows that the advent of the pill has more effect on fertility decline than economic change.

When international family planning began in the 1960s, rapid population growth was recognized as a problem, but no one really knew what the 'solution' was going to be. Some experts wrote of 'beyond family planning', and 'incentives' were discussed. Others said this 'blaming' of the poor and disadvantaged and coercion of the individual, even for the most well-intentioned reasons, was always an unmitigated wrong.

Today, even though some people still fight over yesterday's shadows, there has been a wonderful coming together of those who support family planning as an individual choice, as an effective health intervention and as a way to slow explosive global population growth. Organized family planning programs have already had a profound effect on global population growth. Meeting all the unmet need for family planning could bring the final stable population of the planet to one half of the level it would have been without 30 years of international effort (Figure 16.3). The people have voted: with pills and intrauterine devices and sterilization. People all over the world have demonstrated that they want modern family planning. In Bangladesh, people, of their own volition, want 40% fewer children than the most drastic target of the demographers. Indeed, the unmet need for family planning usually exceeds the demographic 'targets' set by governments. Figure 16.4 compares the demographic targets with the unmet need in twelve countries; a negative number indicates that the satisfaction of unmet need would result in a contraceptive prevalence rate higher than that which would be achieved by meeting the demographer's target.

Family planning needs promotion, just as the soft-drink industry or soap powders need promotion, targeted at individual perception. Most thinking people accept that another doubling of the global population is going to put many strains on the world that our children inherit, but the 'solution' is not to try to persuade people to make decisions for the common good, but to make choices in their own self-interest and for love of their family.

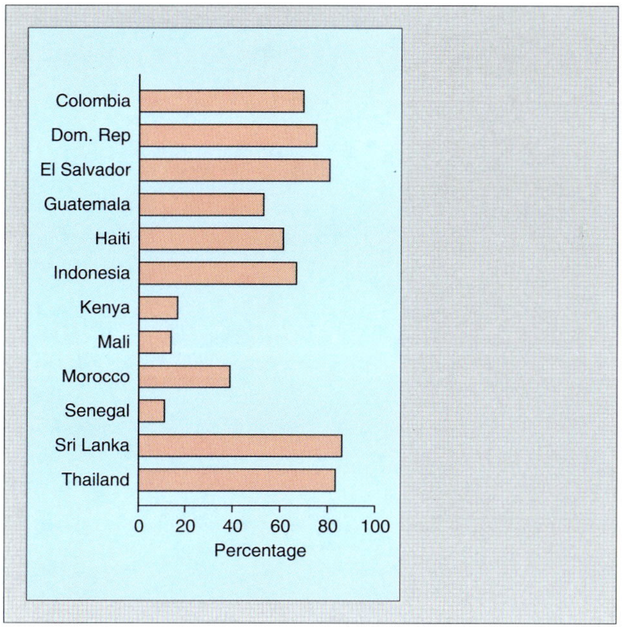

Figure 16.1 Percentage of women with three children who want no more (1983–1987). (Source, Demographic and Health Survey)

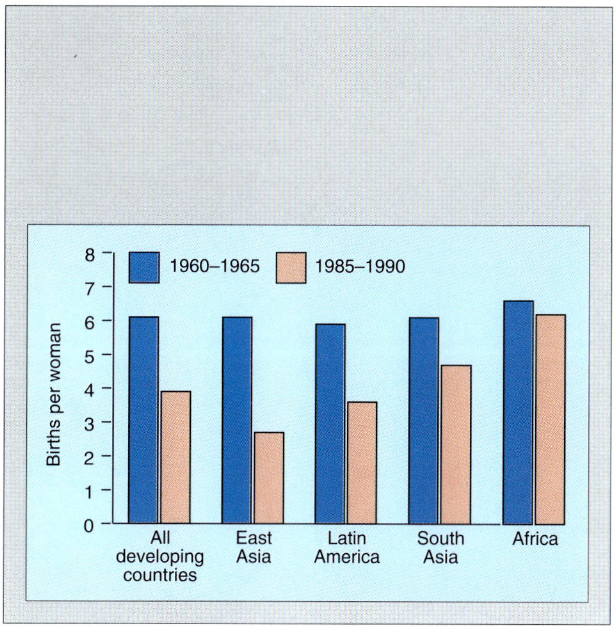

Figure 16.2 Fertility trends in the developing world by region. (Source, *The State of World Population, 1991*. (New York: United Nations Population Fund))

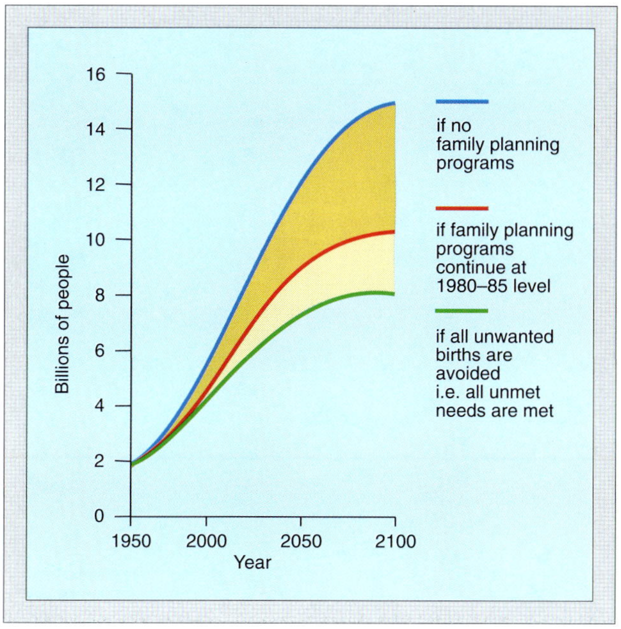

Figure 16.3 Slowing population growth by meeting the unmet need. (Source, *Population Reports*, Series M, No. 10, 1992. (New York: United Nations Population Fund))

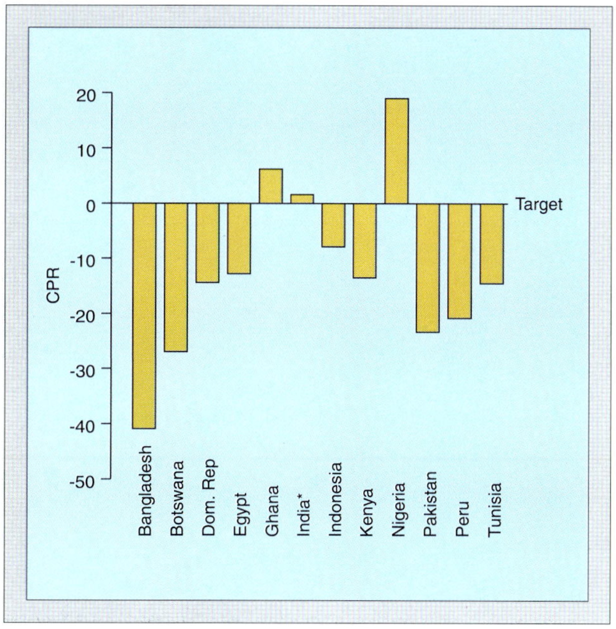

Figure 16.4 Contraceptive prevalence rate (CPR) effect of achieving target vs. meeting unmet need. (Adapted from Senanayake, P. and Kleinman, R. L. (1992). *Family Planning. Meeting Challenges, Promoting Choices*. (Casterton: Parthenon Publishing))

Appendix

International Conference on Population and Development (ICPD)

The International Conference on Population and Development was held in Cairo, Egypt from 5–13 September 1994. The ICPD is the fifth international conference on population. The first was held in Rome in 1954, the second in Belgrade in 1965, the third in Bucharest in 1974; the fourth 10 years later in Mexico City set the population and family planning agenda for the next decade.

The publicity generated by the World Population Conference in Bucharest in 1974 brought population issues to the world's attention for the first time, although the Least Developed Countries (LDCs) took the argument that 'Development was the best contraceptive.' Many governments launched their own family planning programs following discussions at Bucharest and the publication of the 'World Population Plan of Action' (WPPA).

By the time of the next conference in Mexico City in 1984 most developing countries were strongly supportive of family planning programs as ways of improving maternal and child health and reducing population growth rates. The conference in Cairo was the last major population conference of this decade. It set the scene for providing the action-oriented plan to increase world commitment to population and development issues for the next 10–20 years.

The ICPD built on other important international activities as well, including the UN Conference on Environment and Development (The Earth Summit) and the 1993 World Conference on Human Rights. The deliberations that took place at the ICPD will make important contributions to the World Summit for Social Development in Copenhagen and the Fourth World Conference on Women in Beijing, both scheduled for 1995. The ICPD recognized the growing concern throughout the world of the interrelationships that exist between population, environment, resources and development. It also recognized that the women's movement can no longer continue to grow parallel and distinct from the movement towards sustainable development. The ICPD came to terms with the realization that the process of sustainable development is made much more difficult, if not impossible, by the high rates of population growth which prevail when family planning services are not available and accepted.

The document put forward by 182 governments that were represented in Cairo was the Draft Plan of Action for the International Conference on Population and Development. In preparation for the Cairo meeting and this document, three Preparatory Committees were convened. In addition, expert group meetings were convened on six groups of priority issues that were defined as the main themes of the conference; these were: Population, Environment and Development; Population, Policies and Programs; Population and Women; Family Planning, Health and Family Wellbeing; Population Growth and Demographic Trends; and Population, Distribution and Migration. In addition, regional and subregional conferences also provided the opportunity for review of trends and challenges specific to the population situation in different parts of the world.

The main document consisted of 113 pages made up of 16 key chapters.

After a week of somewhat acrimonious debate, the main Drafting Committee of the conference agreed to define the new concept of reproductive rights and laid out a 20-year strategy to deal with the population and development issues.

Underpinning the population issue is the area of contraception. The conference addressed thoroughly the area of contraception. Chapter 12 of the document stated that 'Improved collaboration and co-ordination of activities internationally will increase cost-effectiveness, but a significant increase in support from Governments and industry is needed to bring a number of potentially new, safe and affordable methods to fruition, especially barrier methods. This research needs to be guided at all stages by gender perspectives, particularly women's, and the needs of users, and be carried out in strict conformity with internationally accepted legal, ethical, medical and scientific standards for biomedical research.'

The revised Program of Action received acceptance from the four main blocks at the conference, namely the Muslim states, developing countries, wealthy Western countries and the Vatican, along with its allies. The UN International Conference on Population and Development had a mandate to find ways of curbing world population, which is growing at a record rate of more than 90 million people a year.

The focus was on women – educating them, giving them health and family planning services, ensuring their economic security – and finding the funds to do it.

The action plan sets out an agenda for the next two decades and calls for annual spending of $17 billion by the year 2000 for population control and development, or about triple the current expenditure.

Index